THE FAS

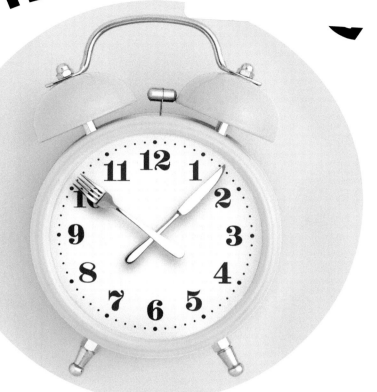

REVOLUTION

getslim

www.getslim.co.uk

Healthy eating plan and recipes created by Sarah Skelton
Designed by Alice Brown
Production director: Sarah Skelton

Printed in United Kingdom

Publisher's notes:
While every care has been taken in compiling the recipes for this book, Digital Wellbeing Ltd, or any other persons who have been involved in working on this publication, cannot accept responsibility for any errors or omissions, inadvertent or not, that may be found in the recipes or text, not for any problems that may arise as a result of preparing one of these recipes or following the eating plan. If you have a low BMI (less than 19), under the age of 18, diabetes, gout, are pregnant, breast-feeding or taking any medications then you should not adopt this style of eating without first seeking the advice of your GP/medical practitioner.

If you have any concerns as to whether this style of eating may conflict with any medical condition you may have then you should seek medical advice prior to changing your eating habits.

About Sarah Skelton

Sarah lives in Norfolk and is CEO of one of the UK's leading online weight loss clubs GetSlim (formerly known as Rosemary Conley Online) and has over 20 years hands on experience in the fitness and weight management industry.

In 1998 she took a complete U-turn in her career after working on her battle to lose weight after having three children by opening up Rosemary Conley Diet & Fitness Clubs franchise based in Norwich helping thousands of men and women to become fitter slimmer and healthier. She re-branded her classes in 2014 and they still run today as Activ4Life.

In 2014 she became the COO of Rosemary Conley Online now known as GetSlim, and in 2017 progressed to the position of CEO of Digital Wellbeing Limited who is the parent company of GetSlim and Healthier for Life.

Sarah has written various weight loss/healthy plans for the online platform, and in addition she has published two books 'Recipes for One, for a healthier you!' and the 'Eat well, Lose weight, Get Healthy' books in 2019.

She is an a accomplished recipe creator and cook who just loves to show people that good tasty food really can be healthy for you.

Acknowledgements

I have loved writing this book as it has allowed me to create something unique but at the same time ensuring healthy eating principles are followed and where no food group is excluded.   The revolution style and format of the days with a reduced calorie intake really helps to reduce the likelihood of complacency which we all suffer from, so it was a real challenge to devise a way that would help combat this.

Creating the recipes and meal formats for this plan has been a form of therapy, I never happier than when I creating new food combinations to share. I find I fully immerse my self in the creative side, so you can trust that every recipe I have devised is created with feeling, understanding and a passion for good tasty food!

Huge thanks must go to Alice Brown, she has worked so hard (as always) on making this book look so good!

And a big thank you to the members of GetSlim and the members of my classes who have tried and tested this plan, I hope you enjoy the journey to becoming slimmer, fitter, healthier and happier!

Contents

The Fasting Revolution

This plan is based on adopting the 16:8 ratio of intermittent fasting combined with reduced calorie intake on certain days to boost weight loss. The unique element to this plan is in the revolutions of the number of days you fast and the calories consumed.

The theory behind introducing a revolution is to stop the body becoming complacent. We are all creatures of habit, often having the same foods for breakfast or lunch, doing the same type of exercise on a specific day each week etc.

When we embark on a new way to lose weight this does not pose problem as our new eating habits automatically kick start our body into accessing our energy stores in a slightly different way and everything works well. However within a few weeks your body has now started to adapt to it's new habits and starts to become less efficient at burning fat and weight loss starts to slow down or plateaus. By applying a revolution pattern the body is far less likely to become complacent and the weight loss will continue at a steady rate.
This theory is not new, any weight-loss expert will tell you that eating different foods and keeping your diet varied is key to a healthy body and promoting weight loss.

The same principle can be applied to exercise, which is why if you ever join a gym they will give you a new fitness plan regularly to ensure the body does not get 'stuck in a rut'

I have just applied all of these principles and my experience to creating this new style plan.

So, what is intermittent fasting?

In simplified terms, anytime that you are not eating, you are intermittently fasting. In real-life terms, we do it every day when we go to sleep for 6-8 hours, we are not eating and therefore this is known as a form of intermittent fasting or everyday life. However, refining this approach to varying degrees has brought about success.

Each day you have an eight hour window in which to eat your meals and then a 16 hour period where no foods are consumed only drinks such as tea, coffee, water and sugar free drinks. You decide on the eight-hour window, depending on your lifestyle. For example it could be 10am – 6pm.

At a basic level, intermittent fasting allows the body to use its stored energy. For example, by burning off excess body fat when the body has no other access to direct energy from food.

The theory is that our body fat is merely unwanted food energy that has been stored away. If we don't eat, then our body will simply "eat" its own fat for energy.

When we eat, more food energy is ingested than can be immediately used. Some of this energy must be stored away for later use. Insulin is vital hormone involved in the storage of food energy.

When we eat, our insulin levels rise, helping our body to store the excess energy in two separate ways. Carbohydrates are broken down into individual glucose (sugar) units, which form glycogen, which is then stored in our liver or muscles. Our body has limited storage space for carbohydrates; and once that is reached, the liver starts to turn the excess glucose into fat. Some of this new fat is stored in our liver, whilst the rest is transported to other areas of our body.

When we adopt an intermittent fasting lifestyle the process goes in reverse. Our insulin levels drop, telling the body to start burning our reserved energy. Our blood glucose levels fall, so the body uses the excess energy stored in our cells.

It is important when adopting an intermittent fasting approach that you:

• Stay hydrated; this includes drinking teas, coffees and low sugar drinks regularly.

- Allow your body to adapt to the new approach – this can take 3-4 weeks
- Cut back on simple carbohydrates, swap to wholegrain, high fibre option
- Choose higher protein based options where possible
- Adopt a healthy balanced way of eating on both the fasting and normal days. Avoid cutting out any specific food groups

With this option you consume your meals within a tight 8-hour window, so the body 'fasts' for the remaining16 hours. In this plan this approach is applied to everyday whether eating a reduced amount of calories or not.
Intermittent fasting is not suitable for everyone

If you have a low BMI (less than 19), under the age of 18, diabetes, gout, are pregnant or breast-feeding or taking any medications then you should not adopt this style of eating without first seeking the advice of your GP/medical practitioner.

If you have any concerns as to whether this style of eating may conflict with any medical condition you may have then you should seek medical advice prior to changing your eating habits.

The Fasting Revolution is great as lost 4lb in first 2 weeks and I have still managed to eat a roast dinner and steak on my normal days, just smaller portions. It was quite easy to get used to 8 hours eating. Pounds seem to be melting away considering I have less than a stone to lose so it really is brilliant.
- Vee A

How does The Fasting Revolution work?

This plan is broken down into a four week revolution cycle. Each week the number of days you fast with a reduced calorie intake changes as does the number of calories consumed on those restricted days.

Once the four week plan is complete, you go back to the beginning – creating the revolution!

Below is the breakdown for the calories on each of the four weeks. If you prefer you can split the total calories across two meals per day or 4 four smaller ones depending on what suits your lifestyle, however, you must stay within the eight-hour window for consuming your foods. You should have the milk allowance each day to help ensure you are getting sufficient calcium for your body's needs.

Week 1:
Four days of calorie controlled fasting, alternated with a normal day.
Each day is 900 calories:
100ml semi-skimmed milk or low-fat plant-based alternative – max 50 calories (milk for tea and coffee come from this allowance)
Breakfast – 200 calories
Lunch – 250 calories
Dinner – 400 calories

Week 2:
Three days of calorie controlled fasting, alternated with a normal day.
Each day is 800 calories:
100ml semi-skimmed milk or low-fat plant-based alternative – max 50 calories (milk for tea and coffee come from this allowance)
Breakfast – 175 calories
Lunch – 225 calories
Dinner – 350 calories

Week 3:
Two days of calorie controlled fasting, these can be consecutive if you prefer.
Each day is 700 calories:
100ml semi-skimmed milk or low-fat plant-based alternative – max 50 calories (milk for tea and coffee come from this allowance)
Breakfast – 150 calories
Lunch – 200 calories
Dinner – 300 calories

Week 4:
1 day of calorie controlled fasting
The day is 650 calories:
100ml semi-skimmed milk or low-fat plant-based alternative – max 50 calories (milk for tea and coffee come from this allowance)
Breakfast – 150 calories
Lunch – 175 calories
Dinner – 275 calories

Week 5:
You go back to week one again.

You will see that there are no set calories to follow on normal days as I want you to think more about healthy options and general portion control rather than continually counting calories, as this needs to become a way of life and not just seen as short term fix.

We need to trust ourselves in our choices, keeping a food diary of what you have eaten will help you do this. It's a great idea to keep a track with photos of the meals you eat as this is an excellent way to see your portion sizes and variety in foods and the diary within GetSlim allows you to do this.

However, over the 20 years I have been in this industry I know that having a calorie allowance brings comfort to many, so for that reason on normal days women should look to consume between 1500-2000 calories and men 2000-2500 per day. I must stress you don't need to count calories if you don't want to, just make healthy choices and you will be fine. Below are some guidelines on portion sizes for normal days to help you get that balance.

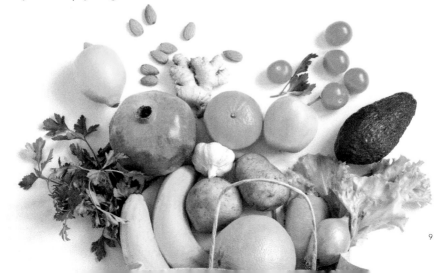

Normal day guidelines:

Either use the following guideline to adapt your recipes. A great selection of recipes can be found at www.getslim.co.uk

Carbs:
- Pasta (60-70g dry weight)
- Rice 55-60g (dry weight)
- Couscous (50g dry weight)
- Lentils/Pulses (50g dry weight)
- Quinoa (50-55g dry weight)
- Sweet Potato(160-180g- raw weight)
- Ordinary potatoes (150-160g raw weight)

Unlimited veg such as: aubergine, carrots, cauliflower, cabbage, edamame beans, fennel, broccoli, kale, leeks, Brussels sprouts, swede, celeriac, asparagus, parsnips, tomatoes, mange tout , peas, sweetcorn, peppers are a great vegetables to bulk up your meals in a healthy way.

Proteins:
- 100-120g beef, lean steak or mince
- 25-30g reduced fat cheese (per day)
- 50-80g low-fat cream cheese, cottage cheese
- 150-160g poultry such as chicken and turkey
- 100-120g lean pork
- 100 -120g lean lamb
- 160-200g any white fish
- 150g any shellfish such as prawns
- 120-130g oily fish such as salmon, herrings, mackerel, sardines etc
- 160-180g cooked weight lentils or chickpeas
- 120 -160g meat free proteins such as Quorn, Tofu, Seitan, Tempeh, Soya, Teff
- 3 medium eggs

The above are the basics, feel free to add home made sauces and or spices to add flavour and change the texture.

Fruit and Vegetables - 5 a day:

You should aim for a minimum of five portions of fruit and vegetables per day (except for ordinary potatoes which are not included within this). Avoid having more than two portions of fruit each day to control your sugar intake. One portion is very roughly equal to 80g in weight. Fruit, vegetable juices and smoothies should be kept to one glass per day – max 150ml to control the amount of sugar consumed.

Eat the rainbow

Eating a mixture of different coloured fruit and vegetables each day will help to ensure that you consume a variety of vitamins and minerals, different types of fibre and carbohydrates – all essential to good health and wellbeing

Red: These fruit and vegetables often contain antioxidants such as Lycopene in tomatoes, anthocyanins found in red berries and ellagic acid found mainly in pomegranate, raspberries and strawberries

Orange and yellow: High in carotenoids: alpha carotene and beta-carotene. Beta-carotene provides the distinctive orange/yellow colour to fruits and vegetables and this is converted into Vitamin A, which promotes eye health and hormone production

Green: These contain the pigment called chlorophyll that gives that rich green colour to broccoli , kale, Brussels sprouts etc.   Dark green vegetables are often rich in vitamin K which helps the blood to maintain normal clotting, however anyone taking anticoagulant medication should refrain from large regular amounts of dark green leafy vegetables for this reason.

Blue/purple: Anthocyanins are powerful antioxidants, which help to protect our cells from damage, and they are also responsible for the blue/purple colours of fruit and vegetables. Purple beetroot is also rich in nitrates that is said to help with blood pressure issues.

White: Anthoxanthins are the pigments that create white or cream colours in fruits and vegetables, and they are found in potatoes, onions, garlic, mushrooms and bananas. It is suggested that anthoxanthins can help to reduce inflammations and promote heart health.

A Guide to Portion sizes for Fruits and Vegetables

Adult portion size is equivalent to 80g.
(As eaten, edible portion, drained weight if canned)

VEGETABLES

Ackee (canned): 3 heaped tablespoons
Artichoke: 2 globe hearts
Asparagus: canned – 7 spears, fresh 5 spears
Aubergine: One third of an aubergine
Beans (cooked) – borlotti, black eye, broad, butter, cannellini, chickpeas, kidney, pinto, soya:
3 heaped tablespoons. Beans and pulses count as a maximum of one portion a day, however much you eat. This is because, while pulses contain fibre, they don't give the same mixture of vitamins, minerals and other nutrients as fruit and vegetables.
Beans (French/green/runner): 4 heaped tablespoons
Beetroot: bottled or fresh - 3 'baby' whole, or 7 slices
Broccoli: 2 spears, or 8 florets
Brussels sprouts: 6-8 Brussels sprouts
Butternut squash: 3 heaped tablespoons
Cabbage (cooked): 4 heaped tablespoons
Cabbage (shredded): 3 heaped tablespoons
Carrots: canned, fresh or shredded - 3 heaped tablespoons
Cauliflower: 8 florets
Celery: 1 stick
Chinese leaves (shredded): 4 heaped tablespoons
Courgettes: half a large courgette
Cucumber: 2-inch/5cm piece
Curly kale (cooked): 4 heaped tablespoons
Leeks: 1 medium leek (white part only)
Lentils: 3 tablespoons. Beans and pulses count as a maximum of one portion a day, however much you eat. This is because, while pulses contain fibre, they don't give the same mixture of vitamins, minerals and other nutrients as fruit and vegetables.
Lettuce (mixed leaves): 1 cereal/dessert bowl
Mange-Tout: one handful
Marrow (cooked and diced): 3 heaped tablespoons
Mixed veg (frozen): 3 tablespoons
Mushrooms: 14 button or 3-4 heaped tablespoons
Mushrooms (dried): 2 tablespoons
Okra: 9 medium
Onion: 1 medium
Pak Choi: 4 heaped tablespoons
Parsnips: 1 medium
Peas: fresh, frozen, canned - 3 heaped tablespoons

Pepper: half a pepper
Pumpkin (diced and cooked): 3 heaped tablespoons
Radish: 10 radishes
Spinach (cooked): 4 heaped tablespoons
Spinach (fresh): 1 cereal bowl
Spring greens (cooked): 4 heaped tablespoons
Swede (diced and cooked): 3 heaped tablespoons
Sweet potato: 1 medium
Sweetcorn (canned): 3 heaped tablespoons
Sweetcorn on the cob: 1 cob
Sweetcorn (baby): 6-8 corn
Tomato puree (concentrated): 1 heaped tablespoon
Tomato: (canned) plum 2 whole – fresh, 1 medium or 7 cherry – sundried 4 pieces
Turnip (diced and cooked): 3 heaped tablespoons
Vegetable juice: 100% unsweetened - 1 small glass (150ml) of unsweetened 100% fruit and/or vegetable juice can count as a maximum of one portion.
It is recommended that we limit 100% fruit/vegetable juices and smoothies to a combined total of 150ml per day (one portion) and consume with meals to reduce the risk of tooth decay.
Vegetable smoothie: 100% unsweetened - 1 small glass (150ml) of unsweetened 100% fruit and/or vegetable smoothie can count as a maximum of one portion.
A portion of unsweetened 100% fruit and/or vegetable smoothie includes 150ml of fruit/vegetable juice; puree; edible pulp or a combination of these.
Government advice is to limit 100% fruit juices and smoothies to a combined total of 150ml per day (one portion) and consume with meals to reduce the risk of tooth decay.
Watercress: 1 cereal/dessert bowl

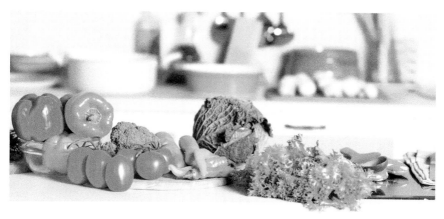

FRUIT

If using dried fruit it's approximately 30g in weight for adults.

Apple: fresh, 1 medium apple or 4 dried rings
Apple puree: 2 heaped tablespoons
Apricots: canned, 6 halves – fresh, 3 apricots – dried 3 whole
Avocado: half an avocado
Banana: fresh, 1 medium banana
Blackberries: 1 handful (9-10 blackberries)
Blackcurrants: 4heaped tablespoons
Blueberries: 2 handfuls (4 heaped tablespoons)
Cherries: canned, 11 cherries(3 heaped tablespoons) – fresh 14 cherries – dried 1 heaped tablespoon
Clementine: 2 clementines
Cranberries: dried 1 heaped tablespoon
Currants: dried 1 heaped tablespoon
Damsons: 5-6 damsons
Dates: dried 3 dates
Fig: fresh or dried, 2 figs
Fruit smoothie: 100% unsweetened - 1 small glass (150ml) of unsweetened 100% fruit and/or vegetable smoothie can count as a maximum of one portion. A portion of unsweetened 100% fruit and/or vegetable smoothie includes 150ml of fruit/vegetable juice; puree; edible pulp or a combination of these. It is recommended that we limit 100% fruit juices and smoothies to a combined total of 150ml per day (one portion) and consume with meals to reduce the risk of tooth decay.
Fruit salad: fresh or canned, 3 heaped tablespoons
Grapefruit: canned, 3 heaped tablespoons (8 segments) – fresh ½ grapefruit
Grapes: 1 handful /14 grapes
Kiwi fruit: 2 fruits
Kumquat: 6-8 kumquats
Lychee (canned or fresh): 6 lychees
Mandarin orange: canned, 3 heaped tablespoons – fresh 1 medium orange
Mango: 2 slices fresh flesh – dried, 1 heaped tablespoon
Melon: 1 slice (2 inch/5cm slice)
Nectarine: 1 nectarine
Orange: 1 medium orange
Passion fruit: 5-6 Passion fruits
Peach: canned, 2 halves or 7 slices – fresh, 1 medium peach – dried, 2 halves
Pear: canned, 2 halves or 7 slices – fresh 1 medium pear – dried, 2 halves

Pineapple: canned, 2 rings or 12 chunks – fresh 1 large slice – dried, 2 rings or 1 heaped tablespoon
Plum: 2 medium plums
Prunes: canned, 6 prunes – ready to eat, 3 prunes – dried, 3 prunes
Raspberries: canned fresh or frozen – 20 raspberries
Raisins: 1 heaped tablespoon
Rhubarb: canned, 5 chunks – stewed, 2 heaped tablespoons
Satsuma: 2 small satsumas
Sharon fruit: 1 sharon fruit
Strawberry: canned, 9 strawberries – fresh, 7 strawberries
Sultanas: 1 heaped tablespoon
Tomato puree (concentrated): 1 heaped tablespoon
Tomato: (canned) plum 2 whole – fresh, 1 medium or 7 cherry – sundried 4 pieces

Reference NHS Choices 2019, 5ADAY Portion Guide

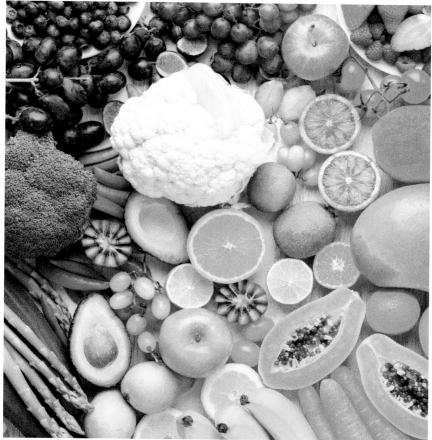

Try to have a rainbow of fruit and vegetables every day!

Fat: Where possible always aim to eat less fat and try to select foods with 5% or less fat content, except for oily fish, oats, nuts, seeds, avocados and some lean proteins. You can quickly check the fat content of most food products by looking at the nutritional information panel on the packaging. Cutting back on fat is easier than you might think. By selecting lower-in fat alternatives you can still eat very well and healthily without feeling deprived. Using spray oils when cooking, such as Rapeseed oil spray means you can easily control the amount of fat used in any meal. Rapeseed oil is incredibly versatile as it can be used cold and in shallow frying without compromise. It contains the least amount of saturated fat of all oils. One to try is Red palm Fruit & Rapeseed oil mix, beautiful colour, great flavour and packed full of good things and it's a fantastic source of Omega 3, 6 and 9. It contains more Omega 3 than olive oil.

Fibre: As adults we should be aiming to eat 30g of fibre per day. Eating this amount of fibre on a regular basis will help to:

• Lower cholesterol levels
• Reduce the risk of bowel cancer
• Helps constipation
• May help to reduce blood pressure through the benefits of reducing cholesterols levels
• Keep you feeling fuller for longer

Finding ways to increase your fibre intake can be difficult, below are some suggestions to help you achieve your goal.

Try to introduce high fibre breakfast cereals into your diet.
• Aim for 5 pieces of fruits and vegetables every day.
  They are low in calories and full of fibre to give that fuller feeling for longer
• Eat fruits and vegetables raw where possible. Boiling can result in a loss of up to one-half of the fibre in the water and consider steaming or stir-frying to retain more fibre.
• Try adding fresh or dried fruit, nuts or seeds on top of your breakfast cereal.
• Add bran to muffins, breads and casseroles.
• Try to have baked, wedged or boiled potatoes with the skin on to be eaten hot or cold.
• Go for wholemeal or wholegrain/multigrain bread instead of white bread.
• Try wholemeal or lentil based pasta, bulgur wheat or brown rice instead of white pasta and white rice.

Remember, brown rice does take longer to cook than white rice so give yourself plenty of time when you first use it.
- Add beans and lentils to salads, soups and stews. Consider beans on toast as a light meal or try some salads with added kidney beans, chickpeas and butter beans.
- Add vegetables to sauces, stews or curries.
- For snacks try fruit or vegetable sticks, unsalted nuts or seeds.

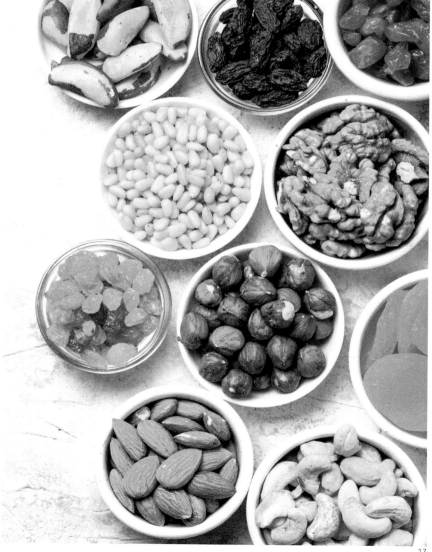

Fluids: We all know we should drink plenty, but actually doing it can be hard.

Adults should be aiming for 6-8 glasses of fluids every day, under normal conditions, which equates to about 2 litres. When we exercise, the weather gets hotter etc. then we need to increase our intake accordingly.

We must hydrate over some time, rather than in bouts as this can overload our kidneys, so consistency and frequency are critical.

It goes without saying that water is the best option for us, and below are just a few reasons why:

• It's cheap; you don't need to buy bottled water, especially in the UK.
• It helps to regulate our appetite
• Improves digestion
• Eliminates harmful toxins and substances, such as alcohol
• Helps to reduce blood pressure
• Contributes to reducing water retention
• Helps to strengthen our bladder function
• Maintains our kidney function
• Helps to keep the moisture in our skin
• Helps to ease joint pain
• Boosts our energy levels
• Reduces the risk of bowel cancer

Research shows that thirst and hunger sensations are triggered together. When we experience a slight drop in our hydration levels, as little as 2%, our brain sometimes sends out a false impression of hunger. As a result, it makes us contemplate eating food when actually what we need are fluids. This is very important, particularly when you are trying to lose or maintain your weight. So, whenever you feel hungry, always have a drink first so that you know your body is getting the fluid it requires to function correctly.
It's not all about drinking water, other forms of fluids are okay too. Tea, coffee, milk, fruit juices and soft drinks are all excellent, although fruit juices should be restricted to 125-150ml per day and all soft drinks should be sugar-free.   Water is also contained in everyday foods you eat, and on average 20% of total fluid intake comes from the dietary intake at mealtimes.

What happens when we started to get a little dehydrated?

Consistent dehydration can cause;
• Constipation
• Kidney stones and gallstones
• Pressure Ulcers

Dehydration can also cause us to become mentally impaired;
• Headaches
• Dizzy spells
• Tiredness
• Reduced levels of concentration and alertness

Tips on how to boost your fluid intake:
• Drink after visiting the toilet.
• Carry a bottle with you at all times to increase access.
• Start your day with a glass of water and a slice of lemon
• Have water with each meal.
• Set goals for the number of glasses you aim to drink every day.
• Every time you drink coffee or tea also drink water.

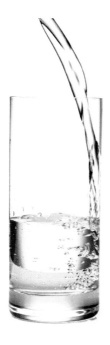
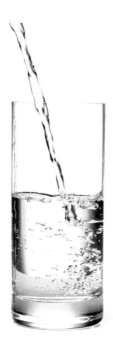
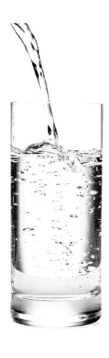

Alcohol: Adults are advised not to drink more than 14 units a week regularly and to avoid consuming more than two units in any one day. It would be best if you avoid alcohol altogether when on a reduced calorie fasting day.

One unit is 25mls of spirits, 75mls of wine, half a pint of ordinary strength lager, cider or beer.

When we drink alcohol, it increases the amount of water we lose from urination, thus resulting in dehydration. This is why if you do drink having a soft drink between alcoholic ones helps.

From a weight gain perspective, it's not just about the energy or number of calories in any given drink. Our bodies are complex machines that can identify certain toxins such as alcohol. Because our body is pre-set to preserve life, it works on excreting the alcohol from our body as quickly as it can. So any food, however healthy it may be, is converted into energy and sent straight to our fat stores, which can result in weight gain. So you can see restricting how much you drink will have a positive impact on your waistline!

Tips on how to reduce alcohol intake:

• Avoid binge drinking
• Use a smaller glass.
• Do not drink on an empty stomach.
• Use low calorie/diet mixers to reduce your calorie intake further and to make your drinks last longer.
• Check the label as many drinks labels indicate how many units are contained.
• Don't eat snacks like crisps and peanuts with your drinks, the added salt will make you want to drink more and may raise your blood pressure.
• If you drink at home, buy a measure so that you know how much you are drinking.
• Keep a drinks diary, as writing this down regularly will help you to determine how much you're drinking.
• Try drinking each drink more slowly or alternating alcoholic beverages with soft or low alcohol ones.
• Have alcohol-free days, ideally three free days per week

Having a drink at the end of a busy day, while cooking dinner or after the kids go to bed is a habit. Habits can be broken, but they take time, and you have to have alternative options in place.

For example, if a Gin & Tonic is your thing, try omitting the Gin or using an alcohol-free gin alternative, using flavoured tonics and still adding your ice and a slice of lemon or lime. You will even get the same feeling mainly if you use the same glass. This is because the eye will fool the brain into thinking its part of your usual habit.

If lager is your tipple, then buy alcohol-free beers, keep them chilled, so you have one ready.

Get out of the habit of drinking because you are stressed or have nothing else to do. Look for other ways to relax. Activities like walking, having a nice bath, reading a can help to distract your mind and feel better.

Remember it is just a habit, and habits can be broken!

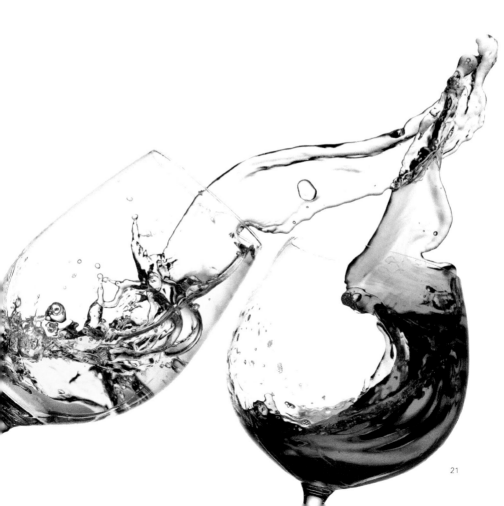

Salt: The recommended maximum intake limit for an adult is 6 grams of salt per day. Salt is also called sodium chloride. It's the sodium in salt that can be bad for your health. Sodium is usually listed in the nutritional information on food labels. Salt is also listed on some foods, but not all.

Salt = sodium x 2.5

If you know how much sodium is in a food, you can work out roughly the amount of salt it contains by multiplying the sodium by 2.5. So if a portion of food contains 1.2g sodium then it contains about 3g salt.

Salt is known to be a contributing factor to High Blood Pressure which it can increase your risk of a Stroke CHD & CV;

There are lots of simple ways to reduce the amount of salt you eat, whether you're cooking, eating out or choosing food at the shops. Take a look at these salt tips to see what you can do.

- Check the label to help you choose healthier breakfast cereals. Try puffed wheat, wheat biscuits or muesli with no added salt.
- When you're buying bread, compare the amount of salt in different types and choose the lower one.
- Try having just a small amount of smoked foods such as smoked meat and fish, or eat them less often, because these can be high in salt.
- Go for tinned veg and pulses without added salt.
- For healthier snacks try to choose fruit or vegetables like carrot or celery sticks, a teacake or a fruit bun. If you are going to have crisps or crackers – check the label and choose those with a lower salt content.
- If you're choosing a ready meal or a ready-made pasta sauce, compare different types and choose the one that is lower in salt.
- Go easy with ketchup, soy sauce, mustard, pickles and mayonnaise - these can all be high in salt.
- Try not to add salt automatically when you're cooking or about to eat. Often people only use salt out of habit.

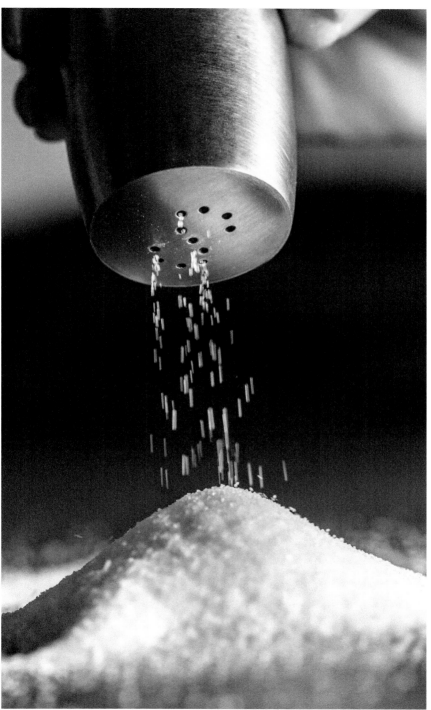

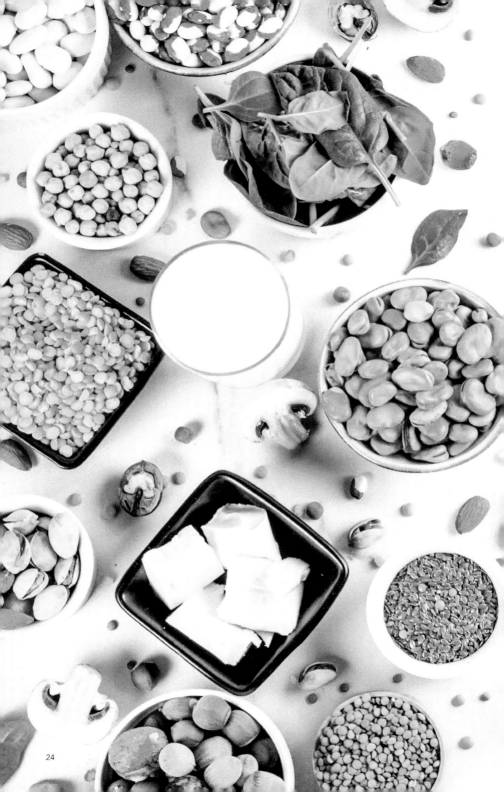

Following a vegetarian or vegan lifestyle?

Being a vegetarian means you live on a diet of grains, pulses, nuts, seeds, vegetables and fruits with, or without, the use of dairy products and eggs. A vegetarian does not consume red meat, poultry, seafood and flesh of any other animal and this also includes omitting any animal by product such as animal fat or gelatine.

What type of vegetarian are you?
There is a variation between one person's interpretation of being a vegetarian to another, and this is due to personal preferences and reasons for following this type of diet.

If you are thinking of becoming vegetarian or following predominantly plant-based lifestyle then it is good to under the various types.

- Semi-vegetarian: excludes red meat but will eat fish or poultry.
- Pescetarian: excludes red meat and poultry but will eat fish.
- Lacto-ovo vegetarian: does not eat any meat, poultry, fish, shellfish or ingredients derived e.g. gelatine and rennet. These vegetarians may also consume dairy products and eggs, but most likely only from free range origin.
- Ovo-vegetarians: include eggs but avoid all other animal foods, including dairy.
- Vegans: excludes all animal products including all derived additives and ingredients.
- Fruitarian: is a vegan, who restricts their diet to only consist of raw fruit and vegetables, nuts, seeds, pulses and grains.
- Macrobiotic: This is a pescetarian diet (sometimes vegetarian or vegan) fixed on ideas about types of food drawn from Zen Buddhism. Its focus is on foods that contain both the ying and yang (based on the Chinese philosophy). With 7 levels that differ and increase in restriction with the lowest level being the most varied which includes fish but still excludes meat, eggs and dairy products. The highest level is based on only consuming brown rice.

When eliminating animal-based foods/products from your diet, there are some specific nutritional elements that you need to consider. The following factors are vital to staying healthy, and they must be integrated into your eating plan.

Iron: Normally we get the most of our iron from red meat, which the body absorbs very easily. However, when red meat is removed from the diet then alternatives need to be sort.

Good alternative sources include:

• Wholemeal bread
• Dried fruit
• Fortified breakfast cereals
• Leafy green vegetables
• Nuts
• Beans and lentils
• Sesame seeds

Vitamin C: Vitamin aids the absorption of iron into the bloodstream. As the body does not retain Vitamin C, you need to ensure you have a food that is rich in Vitamin C in the same meal that contains the source of iron — for example, having a small glass of orange juice with your breakfast cereal, adding peppers or broccoli to a meal. It's important to know that Vitamin C is depleted during the cooking process, so avoid overcooking foods..

Protein: As very few plant sources of proteins contain all the essential amino acids required by the body, except for soya, hemp and quinoa, so it is vital that a vegetarian eats a mixture of different plant proteins to ensure that their nutritional requirements are met.

Good sources of protein for a vegetarian are:
• Seeds
• Nuts and nut butters (e.g. peanut butter)
• Soya and soya products e.g. soya dairy alternatives, tofu, soya nuts and soya mince
• Grains such as wheat (found in cereals, pasta and bread), rice and maize
• Beans, lentils and chickpeas
• Milk and diary products such as cheese, but beware of the fat content, so always choose lower fat alternatives
• Eggs

Another source that some vegetarians may consume is:
Mycoprotein such as Quorn – some variations of this product may not be suitable for vegans, so it is always best to check the label, as some variations contain egg.

Calcium: It is an essential mineral as it helps builds bones and teeth, promotes blood health, and is critical in the function of muscles and nerves.

For vegetarians not consuming dairy products, other sources include:
• Dried fruit: apricots and figs.
• Calcium-fortified foods e.g. soya milk, yoghurts and puddings.
• Sesame seeds and tahini.
• Brown and white bread.
• Calcium-set tofu (i.e. those prepared using calcium).
• Green leafy vegetable: Kale, collard , spinach etc
• Nuts

Selenium: This helps protect cells and tissues from damage.
Good sources are:
• Brazil and cashew nuts and sunflower seeds
• Some fortified breakfast cereals
• Wheatgerm bread

Vitamin B12: Vitamin B12 is only found naturally in foods from animal sources and is essential in helping to build the genetic material of cells and production of blood cells. A vegetarian who does not eat eggs and dairy foods, they should consume fortified foods containing Vitamin B12.

• Vitamin B12 fortified yeast extract, such Marmite
• Vitamin B12 fortified breakfast cereals (with added vitamin B12).
• Vitamin B12 fortified dairy-free

Omega-3: Omega-3 fats are important for good health Vegetarians can get omega-3 fatty acids from other foods sources shown below:

• Chia and Flax seeds
• Oils – Rapeseed and flaxseed – you will see Rapeseed oil is used in many recipes in this book for this reason
• Walnuts and walnut oil
• Soybeans

General tips:

BREAD: Choose multigrain, stoneground brown bread, or rye bread - avoid white bread if possible. If you suffer from gluten intolerance, use a gluten-free alternative. Bread should be a medium slice and one medium bread roll or a slice of bread should be about 35g.

BREAKFAST CEREALS: Choose oat-based or high-fibre varieties, e.g. Jumbo porridge oats, Shreddies, no added sugar or salt muesli or cereals containing natural grains (such as Shredded Wheat and Weetabix). Portion sizes should be 35-40g.

OILY FISH: For good heart health, it is ideal to try and eat two portions of fish per week, ideally one of which should be oily fish – e.g. mackerel, salmon, sardines, herrings. If you are vegetarian, vegan, or don't like oily fish you need to ensure that you eat foods rich in omega 3 fatty acids such as chia seeds, rapeseed oil, algal oil, hemp seed, walnuts, flaxseeds and even Brussels sprouts! Adding chia and flax seeds to your breakfast is one of the simplest ways to achieve this, 1tsp per day will help.

PASTA: Use dry or fresh; ideally brown, lentil or buckwheat based – if not ordinary pasta is excellent. Max serving size is 60-70g dry weight for a dinner.

RICE: Use Basmati rice where possible as this has less effect on your blood sugar levels than regular white rice and therefore helps to keep your blood sugars slightly more stable after eating. Keep your portion size for rice (dry weight) to 55-60g for dinner.

NUTS & SEEDS: Nuts and seeds are fine as long as you control your intake and have just one portion per day – which is about 25g. Brazils, walnuts, hazelnuts are good choices as they contain the least amount of carbohydrates than other nuts.

CHEESE: Use reduced-fat options where possible and control the portion size; no more than 30g of cheese per person per meal.

EATING OUT: Limit eating out to once a week, and choose sensibly. Be realistic and understand that often, restaurants don't have a perfect choice, and that's fine – you are dining out as a treat! Never be frightened to ask for slight changes to a meal, i.e. no sauce, less cream etc. Don't starve yourself before or after the meal, be more active instead and walk an extra 30 minutes the next day.

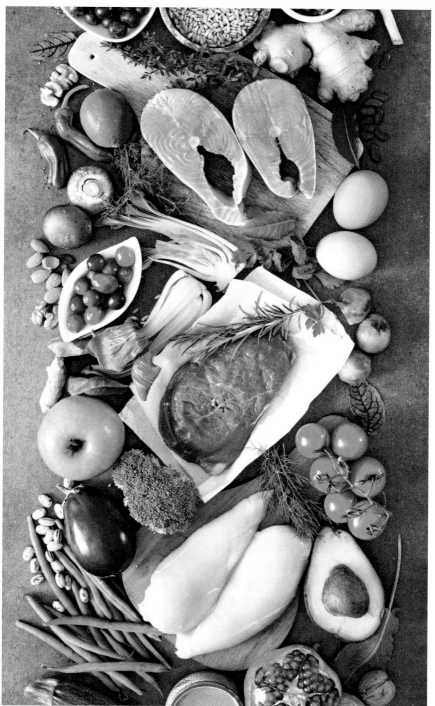

Food shopping tips for a healthier you!

If we want to lose weight or get healthier then we need to make specific lifestyle changes. Since we have the most control over the foods stored in our home, our food shopping habits are essential to the success of our weight loss goals. Small tweaks can make a big difference in the outcome. Below are some great tips to make sure you get the most from your weekly shop!

Plan your meals for the week. Not only does this take the stress out of wondering what is for dinner, but it also means your meals are likely to be more balanced, filling and cost-effective!

Shop with a list. If we got to the shops without a list we are more likely to overspend by buying things they don't want and don't need. A considerable huge amount of food waste is a result of not planning. The list will only work if you use it! The list is no good screwed up in your pocket or at the bottom of your bag!

Don't shop when you are tired, hungry, lonely, bored or upset. When we are emotional we often get enticed into buying things that we believe will make us feel better. It is certainly not good for the waistline nor is it any good for our purse! Sugary and fatty foods become very tempting, as does that bottle of wine or two!

Don't buy just because it's on offer. A deal is not a deal if you don't need it! We can easily get caught up in the buy two get one free scenario. It often leads to eating something we didn't want or need, worse still it may get binned because we didn't use it. Only buy items on sale when it's something that is on your shopping list.

Shop alone. Many people find that when they go shopping with a partner, children or a friend they spend more. Extras appear in the trolley as if by magic and all those good deeds go out of the window. They can encourage us to buy foods that we don't want or need.

Shop at the right time. It might sound strange, but when we go shopping when we are tired, stressed or up against the clock then we look for quick fixes, more processed foods, less good value products and less fresh foods. Choosing a time of day that gives you time to concentrate on the job in hand is crucial.

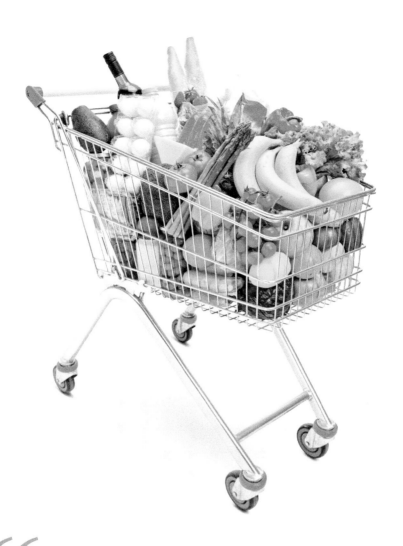

"9lbs off in 4 weeks! - I'm now back within a stone of target! I have eaten a wider variety of foods and the family have enjoyed them too. Would heartily recommend it.. what have you got to lose - except unwanted weight?"
- Gill P

Spices can be kept longer than herbs, although once opened they will deteriorate, it is recommended that you discard them after three months of opening to ensure you get the best flavour. Otherwise they can start to take on a bitter taste or even lose their flavour completely. Always keep your spices out of direct sunlight and seal well after use. The most robust flavours can be achieved by grinding fresh seeds or whole spices as opposed to buying them already ground.

TIP
Warm your spices gently in a frying pan before grinding to release the aromatic flavours. Add at the beginning of a recipe to allow the natural character to develop during cooking.

Know your herbs and spices...
BASIL –lifts any tomato-based dish, try fresh basil leaves

CARDAMOM add the seeds to rice, couscous and curries to give a sweet aromatic touch.

CARAWAY small black seeds used in cakes and great sprinkled on meat for barbecues.

CAYENNE intense heat so use sparingly. Used to dust seafood.

CHILLI use fresh for a strong zingy flavour or dried for less heat.

CINNAMON add whole quills to sauces or use a tiny amount of ground for cakes and puddings.

CORIANDER add to both sweet and savoury dishes. Use in tomato sauces or cakes for a mild spice. Perfect, fresh, ground or in seed form

CUMIN slightly bitter. Seeds need to be fried to release the flavour. Perfect in curries or sprinkle the seeds over potatoes before roasting.

CURRY POWDER use to pep up pasta and rice or add flavour to curries and casseroles.

FENNEL SEED strong flavour of aniseed for pasta, curries and casseroles.

GARAM MASALA great base for curries. Add at the beginning and a little at the end of cooking to give two depths of flavour.

GINGER buy fresh and store in foil in the fridge. No need to peel, the skin is packed full of flavour, and if you grate it rather than chop it you will get more of that lovely natural heat. Great in curries and a great alternative to the heat from chillies if you have someone who is allergic to chilli.

PAPRIKA great smoked added to sausages for a chorizo flavour.

PARSLEY great with fish or in salads

PEPPERCORNS perfect to bring any meal to life. Try red peppercorns for a more subtle flavour. Peppercorns are best used freshly ground

ROSEMARY add to lamb dishes or roast potatoes. Try a sprig of fresh Rosemary in a Gin & Tonic!

SALT – a great way to bring out the flavour of a dish, but use sparingly as we should only have a maximum 6g per day.

STAR ANISE use in mulled wine, beef stews or add to tomato-based sauces.

THYME works well with many meats, tomatoes and Mediterranean style recipes

TURMERIC a great colour enhancer to curries and stews, and packed full of antioxidants too!

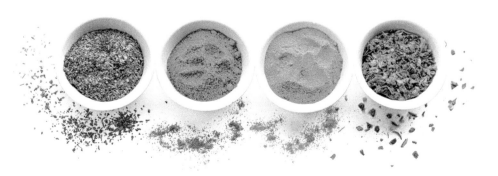

Exercise

Exercise is vital not just to weight loss but to our general health and wellbeing.

Here are just a few reasons why you should exercise regularly.

- Strengthens muscles
- Reduces body fat
- Releases the feel-good hormone, helping to reduce stress, anxiety and depression
- Improves energy levels
- Improves sleep quality
- Reduces the risk of developing type 2 diabetes
- Keeps your bones strong
- Helps to lower raised blood pressure levels
- Helps to reduce cholesterol levels
- Improves lung capacity
- Boosts your immune system
- Boost memory improves cognitive function

Don't panic; this does not mean you need to join your local gym and become a lycra gym bunny! But you do need to focus on making sure you adopt some form of activity into your lifestyle; however busy you are.

With this plan, I've kept it simple; aim for 30 minutes of walking outside every day, everything else is a bonus.

Walking is a fabulous all-rounder; it has an aerobic element (this means your heart and lungs will work a little harder than usual, thus burning fat). You'll strengthen and tone your muscles, especially your leg and stomach muscles. But just as importantly walking outside helps to clear your head, and this helps with those stress levels.

If you can't get 30 minutes in one go, then there is no need to worry. Smaller bite-size chunks spread across the day is perfectly fine too. Getting going: Wearing the correct shoes whilst walking is essential, so choose shoes or trainers that have good arch support and cushioned soles. If you are thinking about more countryside based walking then investing in a pair of walking boots would be a wise decision as they provide more support to your ankles.

Clothing, just wear clothing that is slightly loose and comfortable, there's no need to invest in that lycra! If you are going on a long walk wearing several layers is best rather than a thick top as it allows you to control your temperature more effectively.

As with all exercise, staying hydrated is key as you will need to replace fluids lost through exertion, however large or small that may be. Water is perfect for this and if you are going for a longer walk, may over an hour then a little healthy eating snack would be a good idea to take with you.

If you've not really walked any distance before or are recovering from illness or injury then it's best to begin slowly and gradually. Walking with a friend is a great motivator, making it much more enjoyable and increasing your chances of keeping it up in the long term. Start by underestimating rather than overestimating your capabilities: you'll soon learn how far you can walk before you start to feel tired. Don't push yourself too hard on distance and terrain: the idea is to enjoy yourself, and if you end up too stiff and sore it might put you off going out again. Remember the best activity for you is one that you want to do regularly.

Don't forget, if you have any concerns about your joints (ankles, knees or hips), discuss your exercise plans with your doctor before embarking on a new regime

Level 1 – Health Walk
- Maintain a good posture – stand tall, arms by your sides, and pull your tummy button towards your spine. Keep your shoulders back, down and relaxed.
- Make sure your heel strikes the ground first.
- Let you arms swing naturally at your sides.

Level 2 – Fitness Walk
- Walk with a more purposeful stride, heel down first with toes high, at a faster pace – just below a jogging pace.
- Create a strong push-off from the back foot.
- Elbows are bent at a 90-degree angle and fingers loosely curled.
- Lean slightly forward.

THE PROGRAMME

Weeks 1 & 2
Walk 2-3 times per week, starting with the health walk for a total of 10 minutes and gradually try to increase the duration of your walk, minute-by-minute, ready to go on to weeks 3 and 4.

Weeks 3 & 4
Continue walking 2-3 times a week. Time yourself on the outward journey (walk for approx 8-10 minutes). On the return journey, use short bursts of the fitness walk so that it takes less than 8-10 minutes.

Weeks 5 & 6
Increase to 3-4 times per week. Time your outward journey at 12 minutes. On the first return journey, record your time and try to keep on improving it. The return journey should be predominantly fitness walking now.

Weeks 7 & 8
Increase to 4-5 times a week. Time your outward journey at 15 minutes. Prolong the periods you use the fitness walk. On your return journey, use fitness walking all the way home!

Weeks 9 and beyond
Build up to 5 times per week. You should now be capable of 30 minutes of continuous walking using the fitness walk. If time is short this can be divided into two 15-minute sessions.

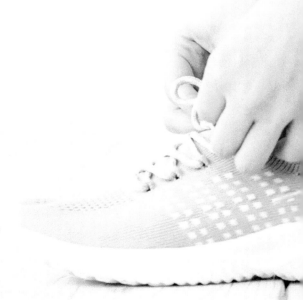

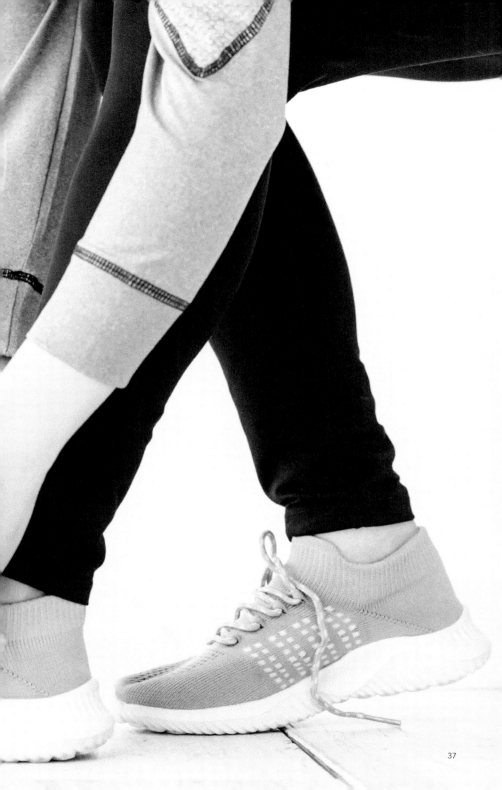

WEEK ONE

2 Weetabix topped with 90g 0% fat Greek yoghurt and 50g blueberries **V**

Mushroom crumpet **see recipe page 57** topped with a small-poached egg **V**

2 small eggs scrambled (using a little milk from your allowance) served with 100g dry fried mushrooms and 1 medium tomato **V**

Porridge made with 45g porridge oats, water and a little milk from your allowance, 1tsp honey or golden syrup topped with 50g blueberries **VG**

Porridge made with 45g porridge oats, water and a little milk from your allowance, 1tsp honey or golden syrup topped with 80g strawberries **VG**

100g of strawberries and 100g of blueberries, mixed with 130g 0% fat Greek yoghurt and ½ tsp flaxseeds or chia seeds **V**

1 slice of seeded bread toasted topped with one medium egg fried **V**

Vegan blueberry, strawberry and oat breakfast smoothie **see recipe page 57 VG**

Egg wrap **see recipe page 58**

Blackberry bircher **V see recipe page 59**

1 Oat, banana and cinnamon cookie **see recipe page 60** plus 6 strawberries **VG**

1 banana, oat and muesli breakfast cookie **see recipe page 61** plus 6 strawberries **VG**

40g Bitesize Shredded wheat with 100ml semi-skimmed or plant based milk (not from your allowance) **VG**

40g All bran with 100ml semi-skimmed or plant based milk (not from your allowance) **VG**

Scrambled egg and mushrooms on toast **V see recipe page 70**

Open egg and prawn sandwich **see recipe page 71**

Large mixed salad topped with 80g cooked chicken

Fennel and spring onion salad with a mustard and honey dressing **see recipe page 72** with 85g baked or poached piece of salmon

Scrambled egg and smoked salmon on a toasted bread roll **see recipe page 73** plus a small green salad

Pasta with pea and mint pesto **see recipe page 74** plus a small green salad **VG**

Pasta with pea and mint pesto **see recipe page 74** plus 6 strawberries for dessert **VG**

Simple zesty chicken salad **see recipe page 75** plus a satsuma or kiwi fruit for dessert

Ham salad bagel **see recipe page 76** plus 1 kiwi fruit or satsuma for dessert

Avocado and quinoa salad **see recipe page 77 VG**

Mushrooms in a creamy tarragon sauce on toasted sourdough bread **see recipe page 78** plus an apple or small pear for dessert **VG**

Strawberry and cottage cheese crisp breads **see recipe page 79** plus mixed salad **V**

Savoury egg, mushroom and spinach porridge **see recipe page 80** plus 1 satsuma **V**

Zesty crayfish and rocket sandwich **see recipe page 81**

Cheese, beetroot and coleslaw sandwich **see recipe page 82** plus 1 satsuma for dessert **V**

Cheese and ham salad sandwich **see recipe page 83**

Pomegranate, chickpea and tomato couscous salad **see recipe page 84**

4 Ryvita multigrain rye cakes topped with 60g extra light cream cheese, 1 apple sliced, a little black pepper and a small green side salad

Cheats sausage jambalaya **see recipe page 109 VG**

Honey and thyme baked salmon **see recipe page 110** served with a large mixed salad

Quick frozen veg pizza **see recipe page 111** plus a small mixed salad

Cheats Chicken Dhansak **see recipe page 112** served with cauliflower rice **see recipe page 128** plus 100g blueberries and 60g 0% fat Greek Yoghurt for dessert

Smoked cod with rice and peppers **see recipe page 113** and 80g cooked broccoli

Pan fried salmon on a bed of wilted spinach, mushrooms and yoghurt **see recipe page 114**

Chinese Style Tempeh **see recipe page 115** served with 140g fresh vegetables (raw weight) stir-fried **VG**

Chicken and Chickpea casserole **see recipe page 116** plus 120g strawberries and 60g 0% fat Greek Yoghurt for dessert

Rich sausage and mushroom casserole **see recipe page 117** served with 220g cooked mixed vegetables (not including potatoes)

Beef and black pudding kofta kebabs **see recipe page 118** served carrot chips **see recipe page 119** plus 120g strawberries or 100g blueberries and 60g 0% fat Greek Yoghurt for dessert

Naan bread chicken and pepper pizza **see recipe page 120** plus a large mixed green salad

Stuffed Aubergine with red lentils **see recipe page 121** with a mixed green salad **VG**

Congratulations
you have completed week one!

Firstly, don't forget to weigh yourself! Hopefully you will find that the scales show a weight loss and also, but just as important, measure your waist, as loss in this area is another great way to measure your progress.

Having started to eat healthily and be more active your sleep pattern and concentration should be improving too. Stay positive and keep up the great work.

This week the focus is on labels. It's good to understand how food labelling works so that you can start to make more informed choices when shopping.

Many food producers have adopted the traffic light system to help you make more informed choices about the foods you buy. This system makes it easier to choose food that is lower in total fat, saturated fat, and sugar and salt. Choose more' greens',' ambers' and fewer 'reds'.

Below is a typical label-

per serving (167g)

ENERGY	FAT	SATURATES	SUGAR	SALT
992kJ	12g	7.5g	4.6g	0.95g
237kcal	MED	HIGH	LOW	MED
12%	17%	38%	5%	16%

of your reference intake
Typical values per 100g: Energy   593kJ/141kcal

For your information
Total fat -
High: more than 17.5g of fat per 100g
Low: 3g of fat or less per 100g
Saturated fat -
High: more than 5g of saturated fat per 100g
Low: 1.5g of saturated fat or less per 100g
Sugars -
High: more than 22.5g of total sugars per 100g
Low: 5g of total sugars or less per 100g

WEEK TWO

1 Weetabix topped with 90g 0% fat Greek yoghurt and 100g blueberries **V**

2 small eggs scrambled (using a little milk from your allowance) served with 50g dry fried mushrooms **V**

Porridge made with 30g porridge oats, water and a little milk from your allowance, 1tsp honey or golden syrup topped with 100g blueberries **VG**

100g of strawberries and 100g of blueberries, mixed with 100g 0% fat Greek yoghurt and ½ tsp flaxseeds or chia seeds **V**

Banana, oat and chocolate smoothie **see recipe page 62 VG**

1 Oat, banana and cinnamon cookie **see recipe page 60 VG**

1 Banana, oat and muesli breakfast cookie **see recipe page 61 VG**

Cheese and tomatoes on toast **see recipe page 63 V**

Strawberry muesli mix **see recipe page 64** topped with an extra 100g of strawberries **V**

Mixed frozen berry smoothie **see recipe page 65 VG**

30g Bitesize Shredded wheat with 90ml semi-skimmed or plant based milk (not from your allowance) **VG**

35g All bran with 100ml semi-skimmed or plant based milk (not from your allowance) **VG**

2 medium hard boiled eggs and 40g fresh baby spinach **V**

Simple zesty chicken salad **see recipe page 75**

Simple minestrone soup **see recipe page 85** plus 1 apple for dessert **VG**

Leftover chicken noodle soup **see recipe page 86**

Super easy broccoli soup **see recipe page 87 VG**

Tzatziki style crispbreads **see recipe page 88 V**

Tuna salad lettuce wraps **see recipe page 89** plus 6 strawberries for dessert

Pearl couscous salad **see recipe page 90 VG**

Pasta with pea and mint pesto **see recipe page 74 VG**

Chickpeas and mushrooms with garlic **see recipe page 91 VG**

Mushrooms in a creamy tarragon sauce on toasted sourdough bread **see recipe page 78** plus 50g blueberries for dessert **VG**

Chunky bean soup **see recipe page 92** and a small bread roll **VG**

Chilli, prawn and apple sandwich **see recipe page 93**

Fried egg with spinach and tomatoes **see recipe page 94** plus a mixed green salad **V**

4 Ryvita multigrain rye cakes topped with 60g extra light cream cheese and 1 apple sliced and a little black pepper

Dinner ideas for fasting days 350 cals:
Mushroom and Marmite spaghetti **see recipe page 122** plus 100g strawberries for dessert **VG**

Naan bread chicken and pepper pizza **see recipe page 120**

Grilled chicken with wedges and roasted tomatoes **see recipe page 123** and 1 kiwi fruit for dessert

Quick bacon spaghetti carbonara **see recipe page 124**

Cheats chicken dhansak **see recipe page 112** served with cauliflower rice **see recipe page 128** and 100g strawberries for dessert

Cod on a bed of smoky butter beans **see recipe page 125**

Butternut squash risotto **see recipe page 126** plus 80g cooked broccoli, spinach or kale **VG**

Sweet potato and okra stew **see recipe page 127** served with cauliflower rice **see recipe page 128** and 100g strawberries for dessert **VG**

Beef and black pudding kofta kebabs **see recipe page 118** served carrot chips **see recipe page 119**

Egg curry **see recipe page 129** served with cauliflower rice **see recipe page 128 V**

Chickpea and apricot tagine **see recipe page 130** served with 100g cooked green vegetables **VG**

Spicy prawn and courgette rice **see recipe page 131** plus 1 small apple for dessert

Minced beef and potato hash **see recipe page 132** served with 100g mixed vegetables not including potatoes

Lemon chicken with fine green beans **see recipe page 133** served with 150g cooked mixed vegetables (not potatoes) plus 100g blueberries for dessert

Congratulations
you have completed week two!

Don't forget to record your weight for this week!

As you know, being active is the key to getting healthier. Have you increased your activity from day one? If not, then now is the time to ask yourself the question, why not? Think about the elements you can improve on. Any positive change, however significant is a step in the right direction!

Maybe plan to meet up with a friend and go for a walk with them, just getting out and meeting people can motivate you to be proactive.

The focus this week is on eating slower. Yes, it may seem a bit strange; however, there can be a delay between physically eating and your brain, recognising that the event has happened and that you are full. When we eat too quickly, we can overeat because the chemicals in our brain that make us feel full have not been activated.

So, eating slower makes a big difference.

If you think about this in a real-life scenario. When you go out for dinner with friends, you will often find that you feel full and struggle to eat the whole meal. This is not always because you've eaten more, but because you have been talking between mouthfuls and your brain is getting those signals and telling you it's time to stop. By eating slower at home, we can replicate the scenario, and we naturally consume less food, but don't feel hungry. By eating the right types of foods, we are unlikely to feel hungry a few hours later too.

WEEK THREE

1 Weetabix topped with 90g 0% fat Greek yoghurt and 100g blueberries **V**

2 small eggs scrambled (using a little milk from your allowance) served with 50g dry fried mushrooms **V**

Porridge made with 30g porridge oats, water and a little milk from your allowance, 1tsp honey or golden syrup topped with 100g blueberries **VG**

100g of strawberries and 100g of blueberries, mixed with 100g 0% fat Greek yoghurt and ½ tsp flaxseeds or chia seeds **V**

Banana, oat and chocolate smoothie **see recipe page 62 VG**

1 Oat, banana and cinnamon cookie **see recipe page 60 VG**

1 banana, oat and muesli breakfast cookie **see recipe page 61 VG**

Cheese and tomatoes on toast **see recipe page 63 V**

Strawberry Muesli Mix **see recipe page 64** topped with an extra 100g of strawberries **V**

Mixed frozen berry smoothie **see recipe page 65 VG**

30g Bitesize Shredded wheat with 90ml semi-skimmed or plant based milk (not from your allowance) **VG**

35g All bran with 100ml semi-skimmed or plant based milk (not from your allowance) **VG**

2 medium hard boiled eggs and 40g fresh baby spinach **V**

Mushrooms in a creamy tarragon sauce on toasted sourdough bread **see recipe page 78 VG**

Chicken and watercress salad **see recipe page 95** plus 1 satsuma

Puy lentil and pearl couscous vegetable salad **see recipe page 96 VG**

Meat free chicken open sandwich: 1 slice multigrain bread, spread with 1tsp plant-based mayonnaise, topped with shredded lettuce, 50g meat free chicken flavour deli slices and 1 pickled gherkin **VG**

1 large mixed salad topped with 2 baked falafels (roughly chopped) and 1 tbs low-fat salad dressing **VG**

1 medium egg, dry fried, poached or scrambled and serve on a slice of multigrain toast **V**

Tuna pate **see recipe page 97** served with 1 slice of multigrain toast

Spicy beans with mushrooms **see recipe page 98** and 1 satsuma for dessert **VG**

Melon, prosciutto and olive salad **see recipe page 99**

Leek, mushroom and pepper pasta **see recipe page 100**

4 Ryvita multigrain rye cakes topped with 60g extra light cream cheese, 1 sliced tomato and 50g sliced cucumber and 6 strawberries for dessert

Dinner ideas for fasting days 300 cals:
Miso honey Quorn fillets with mixed peppers **see recipe page 134** and 130g cooked green mixed vegetables **V**

Tomato and basil mushrooms **see recipe page 135 VG**

Chicken and Chickpea casserole **see recipe page 116**

Beef and black pudding kofta kebabs **see recipe page 118** served with a large mixed green salad and 1 tbsp low-fat salad dressing plus 1 satsuma for dessert

Sweet potato and okra stew **see recipe page 127** plus 120g cooked mixed vegetables (not including potatoes) **VG**

Aubergine, courgette and tomato bake **see recipe page 136** plus 80g strawberries or 60g blueberries for dessert **VG**

Mushroom omelette **see recipe page 137 V**

Mixed bean vegetarian chilli with chocolate **see recipe page 138** plus 1 satsuma for dessert **V**

Mushroom and lemon quinoa bake **see recipe page 139** plus a small green salad **V**

Easy prawn noodles **see recipe page 140** plus 1 satsuma for dessert

Broccoli and cheese pasta bake **see recipe page 141 V**

Lemon chicken with fine green beans **see recipe page 133** served with 150g cooked mixed vegetables (not potatoes)

135g skinless chicken breast (raw weight) grilled and served with 200g any cooked mixed vegetables (not including potatoes)

Congratulations
you have completed week three!

The first few weeks are the hardest, but you have done it! You will be feeling better in your general wellbeing; your vital measurements will be decreasing, and you are a massive step closer to being where you want to be.

This week, think about how and when you say no. Saying no to offers of a sweet or biscuit can be really hard especially if you are offered them when you are feeling hungry. Sometimes we accept out of kindness for fear of upsetting that person or simply because we haven't thought about the impact it can have on us.

The problem is its not just about the extra calories we are consuming but the effect certain types of foods can have on our brain that in turn stimulate us to want to pick/nibble later on. This often happens as a result of eating something rich in simple carbohydrates such as sweets, crisps, biscuits etc.

Preparing for occasions where you are offered food when you're not hungry can help you to decline when the offer comes!

- Think about how you'll respond next time your offered something to eat when you're not hungry
- It can be as simple as saying 'No thanks. I'm ok' or 'I'll pass this time but thanks anyway'
- Enjoy saying no! It's amazing how good you'll feel by saying no to food you previously would have eaten

WEEK FOUR

Breakfast ideas for fasting days 150 cals:
1 Weetabix topped with 100g 0% fat Greek yoghurt and 50g blueberries **V**

1 serving of Mushroom frittata **see recipe page 66** plus 1 Satsuma **V**

Coconut and chia seed with mixed berries **see recipe page 67 VG**

Mushroom crumpet **see recipe page 57**

1 slice of seeded bread toasted topped with 1tsp honey or marmite

Porridge made with 30g porridge oats, water and a little milk from your allowance, 1tsp honey or golden syrup topped with 50g blueberries **VG**

Porridge made with 30g porridge oats, water and a little milk from your allowance, 1tsp honey topped with 80g strawberries **V**

Three pepper frittata **see recipe page 68 V**

Strawberry muesli mix **see recipe page 64** topped with an extra 50g of strawberries **V**

30g Bitesize Shredded Wheat with 100ml of your milk allowance **VG**

2 small hard boiled eggs and 40g fresh spinach

Butter bean soup **see recipe page 101 VG**

Fish soup **see recipe page 102**

Any canned soup max 175 calories **VG**

Edamame and mushroom salad **see recipe page 103 VG**

Indian style roasted cauliflower steak **see recipe page 104** and 1 kiwi fruit for dessert **VG**

Vegetarian stuffed pepper **see recipe page 105** plus green salad **V**

Carpaccio of beef **see recipe page 106**

Meat free chicken open sandwich: 1 slice multigrain bread, spread with 1tsp plant-based mayonnaise, topped with shredded lettuce ,25g meat free chicken flavour deli slices and 1 pickled gherkin **VG**

Large mixed salad, topped with 2 chopped hard boiled eggs and 1 tbs low-fat salad dressing **V**

Quick mushroom pate **see recipe page 107** served with 4 Ryvita multigrain rye cakes and 1 satsuma for dessert **VG**

4 Ryvita multigrain rye cakes topped with 60g extra light cream cheese, 1 sliced tomato and 50g sliced cucumber

2 low-fat oatcakes **see recipe page 149** topped with 30g extra light cream cheese and served with a small mixed green salad V

2 low-fat oatcakes **see recipe page 149** topped with 1 serving of quick mushroom pate **see recipe page 107** VG

Homemade cauliflower pizza crust with mozzarella and basil **see recipe page 142** plus a small green side salad **VG**

Pork and spring vegetable stir-fry **see recipe page 143** served with cauliflower rice **see recipe page 128** and 100g strawberries for dessert

Keralan style fish curry **see recipe page 144** and cauliflower rice **see recipe page 128**

Korean aubergine stew **see recipe page 145** served with 110g cooked basmati rice **VG**

Garlic and rosemary chicken **see recipe page 146** served with 160g mixed vegetables (not potatoes)

120g skinless chicken breast (raw weight) grilled and served with 200g any cooked mixed vegetables (not including potatoes)

Aubergine and chickpea stew **see recipe page 147 VG**

Beef and black pudding kofta kebabs **see recipe page 118** served with a large mixed green salad and 1 tbsp low-fat salad dressing

Aubergine, courgette and tomato bake **see recipe page 136 VG**

Sweet potato and okra stew **see recipe page 127** plus 1 Kiwi fruit for dessert **VG**

Congratulations
you have completed week four!

Well done you are four weeks down the line and you are making positive impact on your weight, fitness and wellbeing.

So what happens now?

As mentioned at the beginning, the reasoning around this plan is to avoid the body becoming complacent and also to help reduce the chances of you becoming bored with your food choices each week - after all, we are creatures of habit!

If you have more weight to lose, then go back to week one and start again. By now you will have understood how each week progresses so you will be feeling more confident about the food choices you make. Start thinking about exploring other options of meal choices for your fasting days.

If you have got to your goal weight, then a massive congratulations! The hard work of maintaining now begins.

For maintenance simply repeat weeks three and four, alternating all the time choosing different days each week to have your fasting day so that your body does not fall into the predictive cycle. If you find you gain a little weight after a holiday then simply add in week two to get back on track!

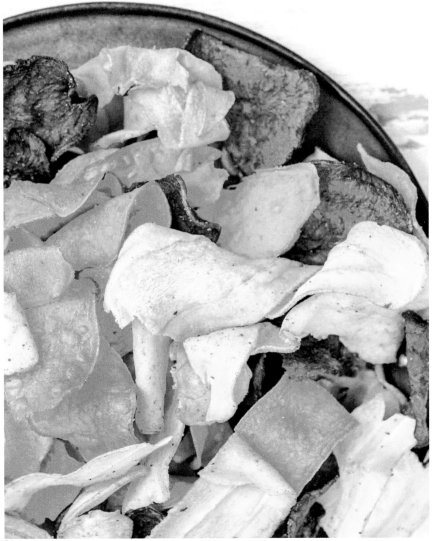

Snacks

It's fine to have the occasional snack between meals if you feel hungry on your normal days. You should not have more than 1-2 snacks per normal day.

1 medium boiled egg
7 Olives
6 Almonds
3 Brazil nuts
4 Walnut halves
1 Low-fat oatcake - **see recipe page 149**
1 Cocoa and raisin energy ball – **see recipe page 150**
1 Date and nut energy ball – **see recipe page 152**
1 Ryvita high protein crisp bread spread with 1 tsp low-fat cream cheese
1 Posh devilled egg - **see recipe page 153**
1 Cloud bread - **see recipe page 154**
1 handful any raw vegetables.
1 portion kale crisps - **see recipe page 155**
1 portion sweet potato crisps – **see recipe page 157**
½ a small avocado
20g reduced fat cheddar
2 tsp hummus with raw vegetables
1 portion spiced baked chickpeas – **see recipe page 156**
4 strawberries
1 small apple
1 small pear
3 dried apricots
3 medjool dates
Overnight slow-roasted tomatoes – 8 pieces - **see recipe page 151**
1 handful of raw vegetables, plus 1 tbsp salsa
2 Courgette bombs - **see recipe page 150**
1 stick of celery filled with 2 tsp of peanut or almond butter

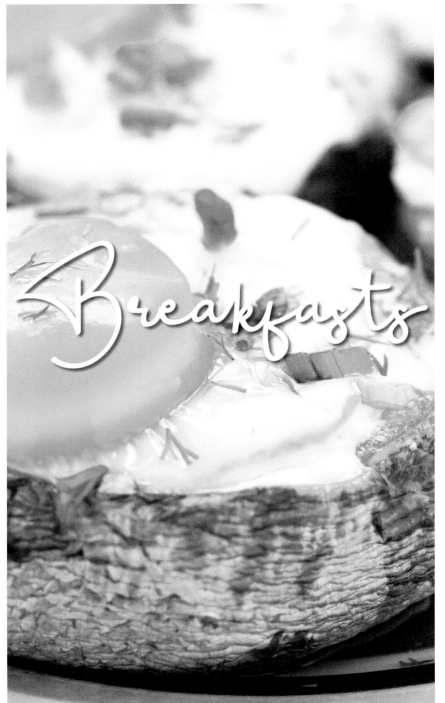

Breakfasts

Mushroom Crumpet

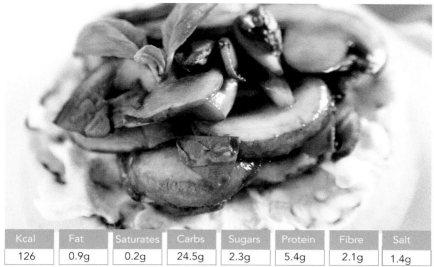

Kcal	Fat	Saturates	Carbs	Sugars	Protein	Fibre	Salt
126	0.9g	0.2g	24.5g	2.3g	5.4g	2.1g	1.4g

Serves: 1   **Prep time:** 5 minutes   **Cooking time:** 5 minutes
Ingredients:
- 10g extra light cream cheese or vegan style cream cheese
- 50g chestnut mushrooms, sliced
- 1 crumpet

Instructions:
Heat a non-stick pan and dry-fry the mushrooms until soft.

Toast the crumpet, then spread with the cheese and top with the mushrooms.

Vegan and Dairy Free Blueberry, Strawberry and Oat Breakfast Smoothie

Kcal	Fat	Saturates	Carbs	Sugars	Protein	Fibre	Salt
201	6g	1g	23.9g	11.1g	10.3g	5.7g	0.51g

Serves: 1   **Prep time:** 5 minutes
Ingredients:
- 15g jumbo porridge oats
- ½ tsps Honea (vegan honey alternative) or golden syrup
- 100g frozen mixed strawberries and blueberries, defrosted
- 200g Alpro plain and unsweetend plant based yogurt

Instructions:
Place all of the ingredients in a blender and blend until smooth. Serve in a glass straight away.

Egg Wrap

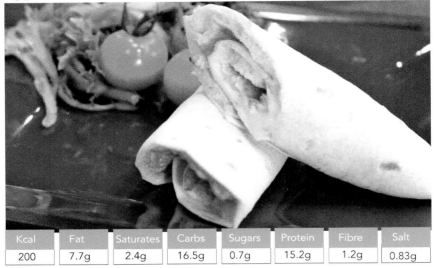

Kcal	Fat	Saturates	Carbs	Sugars	Protein	Fibre	Salt
200	7.7g	2.4g	16.5g	0.7g	15.2g	1.2g	0.83g

Serves: 1   **Prep time:** 5 minutes   **Cooking time:** 5 minutes

Ingredients:
- 1 medium egg
- 1 mini soft tortilla wrap
- 15g low-fat cheese, grated
- oil spray

Instructions:
Beat the egg in bowl. Heat a small frying pan and add two sprays of oil.

Pour the beaten egg into the frying pan, cook for 1 minute then top with the cheese followed by the tortilla wrap and cook for a further 2-3 minutes.

Sliced the cooked egg wrap onto a warmed plate and roll so that the tortilla is on the outside. Cut in half and served immediately.

Blackberry Bircher

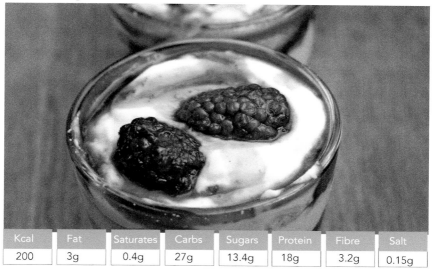

Kcal	Fat	Saturates	Carbs	Sugars	Protein	Fibre	Salt
200	3g	0.4g	27g	13.4g	18g	3.2g	0.15g

Serves: 1   **Prep time:** 5 minutes

Ingredients:
- 1 handful of blackberries, stewed in a little water and cooled
- 140g Fage Total 0% Greek Yogurt
- 20g porridge oats
- 2 almonds, roughly chopped (optional)

Instructions:
In a bowl mix together the greek yogurt and the porridge oats.

Take the yogurt mixture layer in a glass alternating with the stewed blackberries. Once finished leave in the fridge overnight.

To serve place a couple of stewed blackberries on top and sprinkle with the chopped almonds.

Oat, Banana and Cinnamon Breakfast Cookies

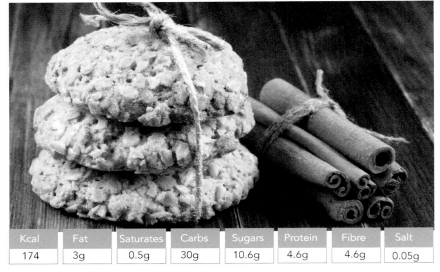

Kcal	Fat	Saturates	Carbs	Sugars	Protein	Fibre	Salt
174	3g	0.5g	30g	10.6g	4.6g	4.6g	0.05g

Serves: 4   **Prep time:** 10 minutes   **Cooking time:** 15 minutes

Ingredients:
- 140g jumbo porridge oats
- 1 large, ripe banana, peeled
- 1 tbsp golden syrup
- ½ tsps ground cinnamon

Instructions:
Preheat the oven to 165C, 325F, Gas Mark 3. Line a baking tray with baking parchment.

In a bowl mash the banana flesh until it's gooey, then stir in the golden syrup and cinnamon. Add the oats and mix until all the ingredients are combined.

Divide the mixture into four equal portions. Roll each portion into a ball and gently flatten until about 1cm thick. Place in the oven and cook for 15 minutes or until firm to touch.

Remove from the oven and allow to cool.

Banana, Oat and Muesli Breakfast Cookies

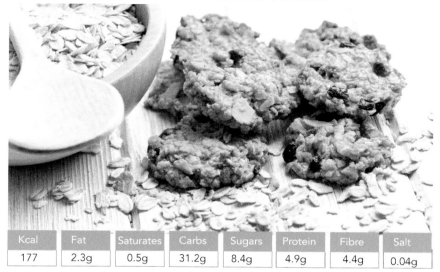

Kcal	Fat	Saturates	Carbs	Sugars	Protein	Fibre	Salt
177	2.3g	0.5g	31.2g	8.4g	4.9g	4.4g	0.04g

Serves: 3   **Prep time:** 5 minutes   **Cooking time:** 15 minutes

Ingredients:
- 1 ripe banana, peeled
- ½ tsps mixed spice
- 50g muesli
- 70g Jumbo jumbo porridge oats, or gluten free porridge

Instructions:
Preheat the oven to 165C, 325F, Gas Mark 3. Line a baking tray with baking parchment

In a bowl mash the banana flesh until it's gooey. Mix in the mixed spice, oats and muesli until combined.

Divide the mixture into three equal portions. Roll each portion into a ball and gently flatten until about 1cm thick. Place in the oven and cook for 15 minutes or until firm to touch.

Remove from the oven and allow to cool. These will keep for up to 5 days in an airtight container.

Banana, Oat and Chocolate Smoothie

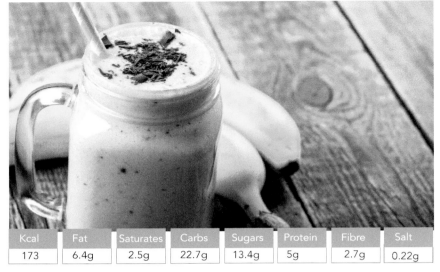

Kcal	Fat	Saturates	Carbs	Sugars	Protein	Fibre	Salt
173	6.4g	2.5g	22.7g	13.4g	5g	2.7g	0.22g

Serves: 2   **Prep time:** 5 minutes

Ingredients:
- 25g Jumbo porridge oats
- 320ml unsweetened oat milk
- 1 large, ripe banana, peeled and roughly chopped
- 20g cocoa powder

Instructions:
Place all of the ingredients into a blender and blitz until smooth

Pour into two glasses, and grate over the dark chocolate if using. Serve straight away.

Cheese and Tomatoes on Toast

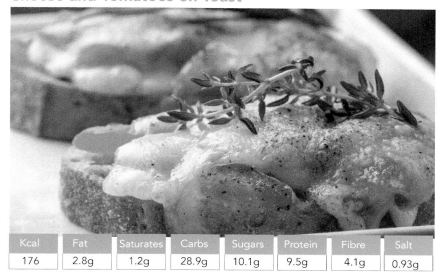

Kcal	Fat	Saturates	Carbs	Sugars	Protein	Fibre	Salt
176	2.8g	1.2g	28.9g	10.1g	9.5g	4.1g	0.93g

Serves: 2   **Prep time:** 5 minutes   **Cooking time:** 10 minutes

Ingredients:
- 1x400g can plum tomatoes
- 2 tsps Worcestershire sauce
- 20g reduced-fat or low-fat mature cheese, grated
- 2 slices multigrain bread

Instructions:
Heat the tomatoes in a small saucepan.

Toast the bread lightly on both sides under a hot grill.

Place the toasted bread on a baking tray and cover with the tomatoes. Sprinkle with Worcestershire sauce and top with grated cheese. Return to the grill for 1-2 minutes until the cheese starts to melt.

TIP
You can use overripe chopped fresh tomatoes instead of canned tomatoes.

Strawberry Muesli Mix

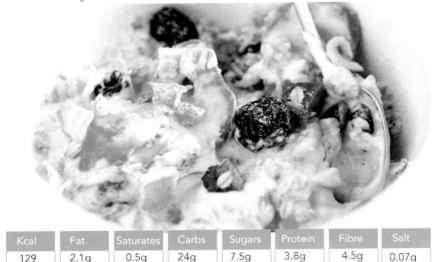

Kcal	Fat	Saturates	Carbs	Sugars	Protein	Fibre	Salt
129	2.1g	0.5g	24g	7.5g	3.8g	4.5g	0.07g

Serves: 1   **Prep time:** 10 minutes

Ingredients:
- 1 tbsp low-fat yoghurt
- 30g reduced sugar muesli
- 50g fresh strawberries
- 2 tbsps water, boiling, from a kettle

Instructions:

Measure the muesli into a bowl. Pour the boiling water over and allow to stand while you prepare the strawberries.

Wash and hull the strawberries and slice into the muesli.

Mix in the yogurt, and serve.

TIP

You can substitute the strawberries for any other berries of your choice.

Mixed Frozen Berry Smoothie

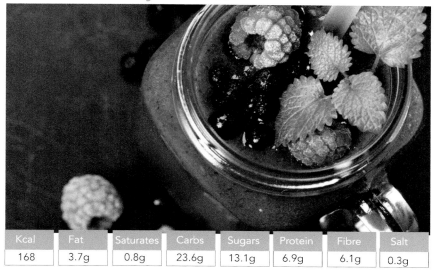

Kcal	Fat	Saturates	Carbs	Sugars	Protein	Fibre	Salt
168	3.7g	0.8g	23.6g	13.1g	6.9g	6.1g	0.3g

Serves: 1   **Prep time:** 5 minutes

Ingredients:

- 125g frozen mixed berries
- 120ml almond milk or soya milk
- 80g reduced-fat dairy free yoghurt
- 10g jumbo porridge oats

Instructions:

Place all of the ingredients into a blender and blitz until smooth.

Serve straight away

Mushroom Frittata

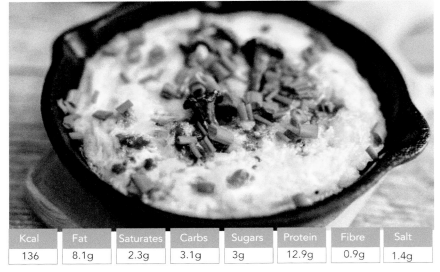

Kcal	Fat	Saturates	Carbs	Sugars	Protein	Fibre	Salt
136	8.1g	2.3g	3.1g	3g	12.9g	0.9g	1.4g

Serves: 2   **Prep time:** 5 minutes   **Cooking time:** 10 minutes

Ingredients:
- 1 tbsp tamari gluten free soy sauce or light soy sauce
- 225g (8oz) chestnut mushrooms, sliced
- black pepper, freshly ground
- 3 eggs
- 2 tbsps skimmed milk
- 4 spring onions, finely chopped

Instructions:
Finely slice the spring onions, reserving a tablespoon for decoration. Preheat a non stick frying pan. Add the mushrooms and spring onions and dry fry for 2-3 minutes until lightly coloured, seasoning well with black pepper.

In a mixing bowl, whisk the eggs, gradually adding the milk and soy sauce. Pour the mixture into the pan, reduce the heat and cook gently until the frittata is just set, scatter over the remaining spring onions. Slide on to a warmed plate. Divide in two.

Coconut and Chia Seed with Mixed Berries

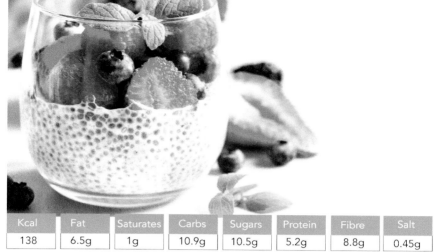

Kcal	Fat	Saturates	Carbs	Sugars	Protein	Fibre	Salt
138	6.5g	1g	10.9g	10.5g	5.2g	8.8g	0.45g

Serves: 1   **Prep time:** 5 minutes plus 1-2 hours standing time

Ingredients:
- 160g canned coconut milk
- 50g mixed fresh berries
- 1 ½ tbsp's chia seeds
- Dash of vanilla extract

Instructions:
Mix the coconut milk, vanilla and chia seeds together and pour into a tumbler. Leave to thicken for 1-2 hours in the fridge or for better results overnight.

Just before serving top with the mixed berries.

TIP
This makes a perfect breakfast too!

Three Pepper Frittata

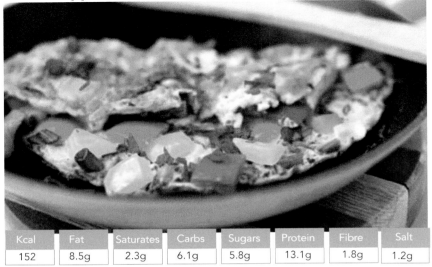

Kcal	Fat	Saturates	Carbs	Sugars	Protein	Fibre	Salt
152	8.5g	2.3g	6.1g	5.8g	13.1g	1.8g	1.2g

Serves: 2   **Prep time:** 5 minutes   **Cooking time:** 10 minutes

Ingredients:
- ½ red pepper and green pepper and yellow pepper, seeded and diced
- 1 tbsp parsley, finely chopped
- black pepper, freshly ground
- 3 eggs
- 2 tbsps skimmed milk
- 1 tbsp light soy sauce

Instructions:

Preheat a non-stick frying pan, add the peppers and dry-fry for 2-3 minutes until lightly coloured, seasoning well with black pepper.

In a mixing bowl, whisk the eggs and gradually add the milk, parsley and soy sauce.

Pour the mixture into the frying pan, reduce the heat and cook gently until the frittata is just set.

Fold the frittata in half and slide on to a warmed serving plate. Serve with grilled tomatoes and a mixed salad.

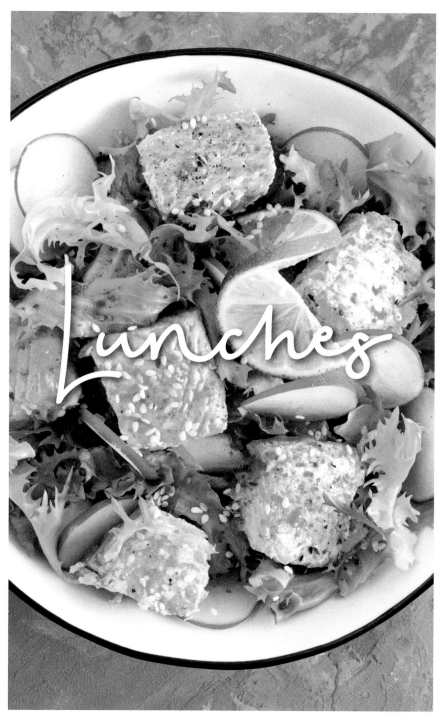

Lunches

Scrambled Egg and Mushrooms on Bread

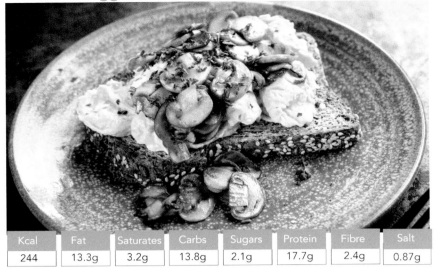

Kcal	Fat	Saturates	Carbs	Sugars	Protein	Fibre	Salt
244	13.3g	3.2g	13.8g	2.1g	17.7g	2.4g	0.87g

Serves: 1   **Prep time:** 5 minutes   **Cooking time:** 10 minutes

Ingredients:
- 2 medium sized eggs
- 80g button mushrooms, cleaned and thinly sliced
- 1 slice seeded bread
- Worcestershire sauce
- Rapeseed oil spray

Instructions:
In a small bowl crack the eggs and add the milk and beat lightly with a fork

Preheat a small frying pan and add a couple of sprays of the rapeseed oil and add the mushrooms. Cook for 4-5 minutes until softened and starting to go brown. Add a few drops of Worcestershire sauce and stir to combine then transfer the mushrooms to a warmed plate.

Using the same frying pan, re-heat gently and add the milk and egg mixture. Cook gently stirring all the time until the mixture has scrambled.

Place the bread on a warmed plate and top with the scrambled egg and cooked mushrooms. Serve straight away

Open Egg and Prawn Sandwich

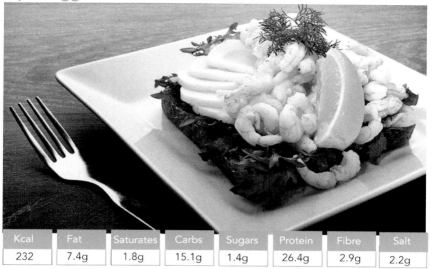

Kcal	Fat	Saturates	Carbs	Sugars	Protein	Fibre	Salt
232	7.4g	1.8g	15.1g	1.4g	26.4g	2.9g	2.2g

Serves: 1   **Prep time:** 5 minutes   **Cooking time:** 10 minutes

Ingredients:

- 100g cooked peeled prawns
- 1 egg, hard-boiled and cooled
- 1 handful salad leaves
- 2 tsps extra light mayonaise
- 1 wedge of lemon, to garnish, optional

Instructions:

Spread the mayonnaise over one side of the slice of bread and top with the salad leaves.

Peel and slice the hard-boiled egg and arrange that over the salad leaves. Sprinkle over the prawns and serve.

Optional - squeeze over a little fresh lemon juice just before eating.

Fennel and Spring Onion Salad with a Mustard and Honey Dressing

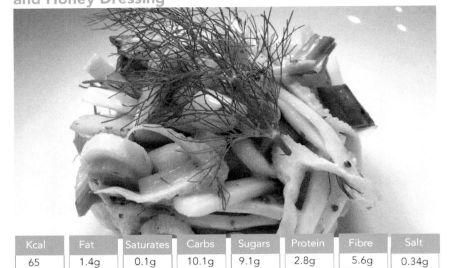

Kcal	Fat	Saturates	Carbs	Sugars	Protein	Fibre	Salt
65	1.4g	0.1g	10.1g	9.1g	2.8g	5.6g	0.34g

Serves: 1   **Prep time:** 5 minutes

Ingredients:
- 2 spring onions
- 1 fennel bulb
- 1 tsp extra light mayonaise
- 1 tsp honey
- 1 tsp white wine vinegar
- ½ tsps wholegrain mustard

Instructions:

Clean the fennel bulb and slice, reserving a few of the fronds for the garnish. Then clean and slice the spring onions.

In a bowl add the wholegrain mustard, mayonnaise, honey and white wine vinegar and mix until combined

Add the sliced fennel and spring onions to the dressing and stir gently to coat evenly in the sauce. Serve straight away

Scrambled and smoked Salmon on a Toasted Bread Roll

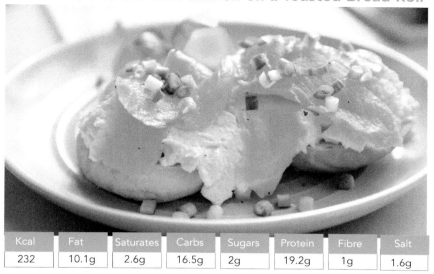

Kcal	Fat	Saturates	Carbs	Sugars	Protein	Fibre	Salt
232	10.1g	2.6g	16.5g	2g	19.2g	1g	1.6g

Serves: 1   **Prep time:** 5 minutes   **Cooking time:** 10 minutes

Ingredients:
- 1x30g soft bread roll
- 35g smoked salmon
- 1 medium egg
- 1 tbsp semi-skimmed milk
- 1 spring onion, cleaned, root removed and sliced
- freshly ground black pepper

Instructions:
Pre-heat the grill. Cut the bread roll in half and gently toast cut side up under the grill until golden brown.

Crack the egg into a small saucepan and add the milk and a little black pepper if using and beat with a wooden spoon. Place the pan onto a medium heat and cook the egg and milk mixture until it starts to scramble, stirring all the time until any residue liquid is absorbed. Remove from the heat.

Place the toasted bread onto a plate top with the scrambled egg, then the smoke salmon and finally sprinkle over the sliced spring onion if using and serve straight away.

Pasta with Pea and Mint Pesto

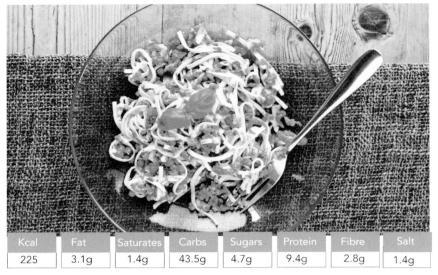

Kcal	Fat	Saturates	Carbs	Sugars	Protein	Fibre	Salt
225	3.1g	1.4g	43.5g	4.7g	9.4g	2.8g	1.4g

Serves: 2   **Prep time:** 5 minutes   **Cooking time:** 20 minutes

Ingredients:
- 2 spring onions, cleaned, root removed and finely chopped
- 100g frozen peas
- 80ml water
- ½ tsps ground coriander
- 2 tsps fresh mint
- 2 tsps half-fat creme fraiche
- 100g dry pasta linguine
- 1 vegetable stock cube
- salt and freshly ground black pepper

Instructions:

Place the spring onions, garlic and peas in a small saucepan with the water. Simmer gently for 2 minutes. Allow to cool slightly then pour into a food processor adding the coriander, mint and crème fraîche and blitz together for a few minutes.

Meanwhile, cook the pasta in a pan of water containing the stock cube. Strain the pasta well, return to the pan and add the sauce and toss well. Serve straight away with a mixed salad

Simple Zesty Chicken Salad

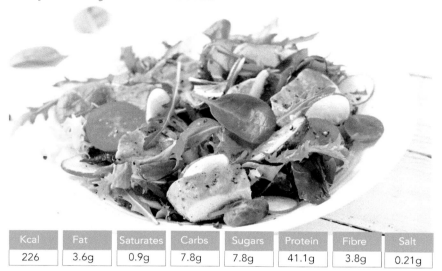

Kcal	Fat	Saturates	Carbs	Sugars	Protein	Fibre	Salt
226	3.6g	0.9g	7.8g	7.8g	41.1g	3.8g	0.21g

Serves: 1   **Prep time:** 5 minutes

Ingredients:

- 120g cooked chicken breast, skinned removed before cooking and cubed
- 1x4cm piece of cucumber, sliced
- 8 cherry tomatoes, halved
- 3 radishes, trimmed and sliced
- juice and zest of 1 lime
- freshly ground black pepper

Instructions:

Place the lime juice and zest in a mixing bowl and add a generous amount of freshly ground black pepper. Lightly mix to make a dressing. Add the salad leaves, tomatoes, radishes and cucumber to the dressing and toss until evenly coated

Transfer the salad to a large plate and top with the cubes of chicken. Serve straight away or store in the fridge for up to 4 hours.

Ham Salad Bagel

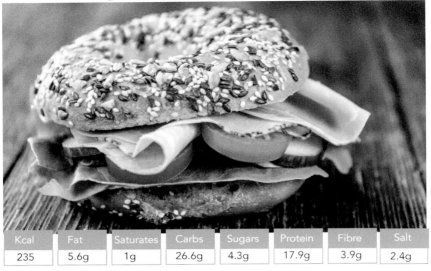

Kcal	Fat	Saturates	Carbs	Sugars	Protein	Fibre	Salt
235	5.6g	1g	26.6g	4.3g	17.9g	3.9g	2.4g

Serves: 1   **Prep time:** 5 minutes
Ingredients:
- 1x60g Warburtons Protein seeded bagel
- 50g sliced ham
- 2 lettuce leaves
- 1x2cm piece of cucumber, sliced
- 1 small ripe tomato, sliced
- ¼ tsps wholegrain mustard
- 1 ½ tsps extra light mayonaise

Instructions:
Mix the mayonnaise and mustard together in a small bowl. Cut the bagel in half and spread the dressing equally with the mustard dressing.

Add the remaining ingredients to the bottom piece of the bagel by layering them - starting with the lettuce at the bottom. Place the top of the bagel on top and eat straight away or wrap in cling film and keep in the fridge for up to 24 hours

Avocado and Quinoa Salad

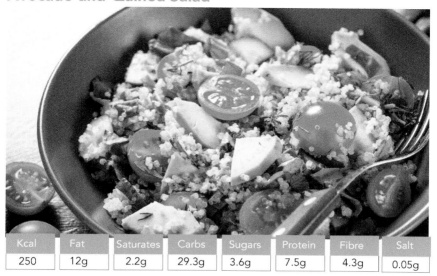

Kcal	Fat	Saturates	Carbs	Sugars	Protein	Fibre	Salt
250	12g	2.2g	29.3g	3.6g	7.5g	4.3g	0.05g

Serves: 2   **Prep time:** 10 minutes

Ingredients:
- 1 tsp fresh dill, chopped or ¼ tsps dried dill
- 20g baby leaf spinach, washed and dried
- salt and freshly ground black pepper
- juice of one lime
- 4cm piece of cucumber, cut into chunks
- 8 cherry tomatoes, halved
- ½ small avocado, peeled, stone removed and diced
- 245g cooked quinoa

Instructions:

Place all the ingredients except the spinach and the salt and pepper into a bowl and toss until evenly mixed and coated in the lime juice and dill. Season with the salt and black pepper

Tear the spinach leaves in half and place in a serving bowl. Top with the avocado and quinoa salad and serve straight away

Mushrooms in a Creamy Tarragon Sauce on Toasted Sourdough Bread

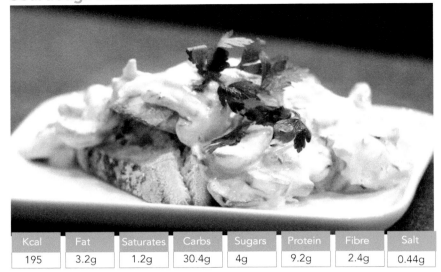

Kcal	Fat	Saturates	Carbs	Sugars	Protein	Fibre	Salt
195	3.2g	1.2g	30.4g	4g	9.2g	2.4g	0.44g

Serves: 1   **Prep time:** 5 minutes   **Cooking time:** 10 minutes

Ingredients:
- 130g mixed fresh mushrooms, cleaned and sliced
- 1 ½ tbsps low-fat cream cheese or vegan style cream cheese
- freshly ground black pepper, optional
- Rapeseed oil spray
- 1 tbsp semi-skimmed milk or unsweetend soya milk or unsweetend oat milk
- 40g sourdough bread or gluten free sourdough bread, cut into two slices
- 1 tbsp fresh tarragon, roughly chopped

Instructions:
Heat a small frying pan and add a couple of sprays of the rapeseed oil. Add the spring onions and the sliced mushrooms and cook for 3-4 minutes or until softened

Add the tarragon to the frying pan and stir in, Reduce the heat and add the cream cheese followed by the milk, stir continuously until the sauce is smooth.

Toast the sourdough bread and place on a small warmed plate. Gently our over the creamy mushroom mixture, season with a little black pepper if you wish and serve straight away.

Strawberry and Cottage Cheese Crispbreads

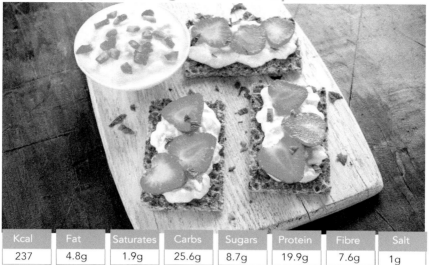

Kcal	Fat	Saturates	Carbs	Sugars	Protein	Fibre	Salt
237	4.8g	1.9g	25.6g	8.7g	19.9g	7.6g	1g

Serves: 1   **Prep time:** 5 minutes

Ingredients:
- 2 fresh mint leaves, chopped (optional)
- 3 multigrain rye crispbreads, such as Ryvita
- 150g low-fat natural cottage cheesee

Instructions:

Divide the cottage cheese equally and evenly between the three crispbreads.

Top with the sliced strawberries and sprinkle over the fresh mint if using. Serve straight away.

TIP

You can swap the mint for freshly ground black pepper

Savoury Egg, Mushroom and Spinach Porridge

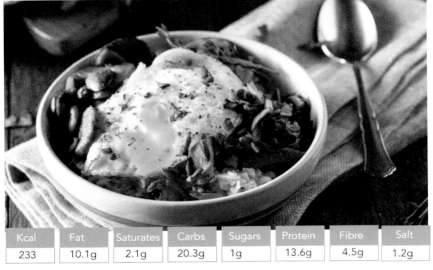

Kcal	Fat	Saturates	Carbs	Sugars	Protein	Fibre	Salt
233	10.1g	2.1g	20.3g	1g	13.6g	4.5g	1.2g

Serves: 1   **Prep time:** 2 minutes   **Cooking time:** 8 minutes

Ingredients:
- 35g jumbo porridge oats
- 200ml vegetable stock
- 1 medium egg
- 60g chestnut mushrooms, cleaned and sliced
- 25g spinach leaves, sliced
- black pepper
- Rapeseed oil spray

Instructions:
Put the porridge oats in a saucepan, and pour in the vegetable stock. Bring to the boil and simmer for 4-5 minutes, stirring from time to time and watching carefully that it doesn't stick to the bottom of the pan.

Whilst the porridge is cooking heat a small frying pan and add a couple of sprays of the rapeseed oil and add the mushrooms and cook for 1-2 minutes. Move the mushrooms to the side and add one more spray of the oil and crack the egg into the pan, gently fry for 3-4 minutes taking care not to over-cook the egg.

Remove the porridge from the heat and transfer to a warmed bowl. Topped with chopped spinach leaves, mushrooms and a fried egg.

Season with a little black pepper and serve straight away.

Zesty Crayfish and Rocket Sandwich

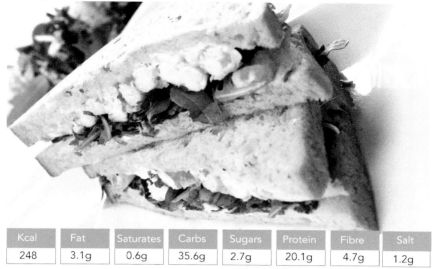

Kcal	Fat	Saturates	Carbs	Sugars	Protein	Fibre	Salt
248	3.1g	0.6g	35.6g	2.7g	20.1g	4.7g	1.2g

Serves: 1   **Prep time:** 5 minutes

Ingredients:
- 80g cooked crayfish tails
- 2– medium slices of granary bread
- 20g rocket leaves, or any salad leaves
- 2 tsps extra light mayonaise
- zest and juice of 1 small lime
- freshly ground black pepper

Instructions:
Place the mayonnaise in a small bowl and add the lime juice, zest and a little freshly ground black pepper, mix together to make a dressing.

Spread the dressing over the top of the two slices of granary bread. Top one slice of bread with the crayfish and the rocket, top with the remaining slice of bread and cut in half. Serve straight away or cover in clingfilm and store in the fridge for up to 24 hours.

TIP
You can swap the crayfish for cooked peeled prawns

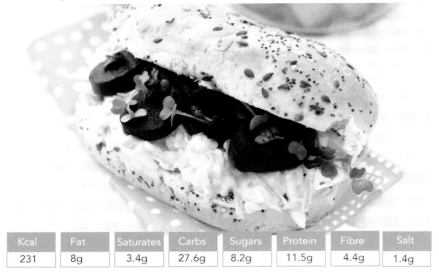

Kcal	Fat	Saturates	Carbs	Sugars	Protein	Fibre	Salt
231	8g	3.4g	27.6g	8.2g	11.5g	4.4g	1.4g

Serves: 1   **Prep time:** 5 minutes

Ingredients:
- 1 multiseed roll or 1 gluten free multiseeded bread roll
- salt and black pepper
- 1 tbsp carrot, grated
- 1 tbsp mayonnaise
- 1 spring onion, finely chopped
- 2 baby beetroots, sliced
- 25g reduced-fat or low-fat mature cheese, grated

Instructions:

Split a multiseed roll in half using a sharp knife. Mix together 1 tbsp mayonnaise, 1 tbsp grated carrot and 1 finely chopped spring onion, seasoning with salt and black pepper.

Spread the mixture on both sides of the roll. Add 15g grated low-fat mature cheese and 2 sliced baby beetroots. Press both sides of the roll together and cut in half. Wrap with food wrap until ready to eat.

TIP

Transform a simple cheese sandwich with the sweetness of beetroot. Perfect for work or school pack lunches!

Cheese and Ham Salad Sandwich

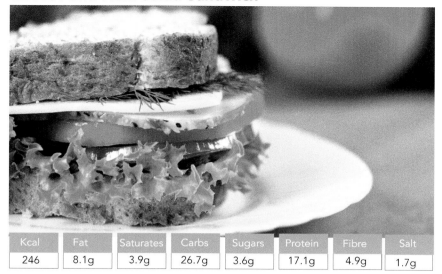

Kcal	Fat	Saturates	Carbs	Sugars	Protein	Fibre	Salt
246	8.1g	3.9g	26.7g	3.6g	17.1g	4.9g	1.7g

Serves: 1   **Prep time:** 5 minutes

Ingredients:

- 30g slice of lean cooked ham
- 25g slice of reduced-fat Cheddar cheese
- 1 handful of mixed salad (lettuce, sliced tomato, onion etc)
- 2 tsps extra light mayonaise
- 2 slices medium thickness wholemeal bread

Instructions:

Spread one side of each of the slices of bread with the mayonnaise

Lay the salad on top of one of the slices of bread (mayonnaise side up), top with the cheese and ham and the final slice or bread

Serve straight away or store in the refridgerator for 24 hours

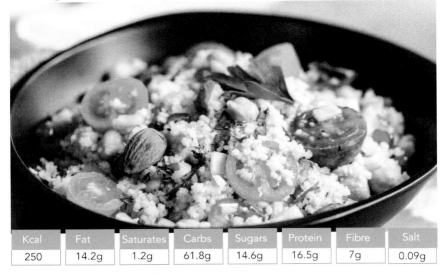

Kcal	Fat	Saturates	Carbs	Sugars	Protein	Fibre	Salt
250	14.2g	1.2g	61.8g	14.6g	16.5g	7g	0.09g

Serves: 2   **Prep time:** 15 minutes

Ingredients:
- 145ml boiling water
- 50g dry couscous
- Juice from one lemon
- pinch of salt
- 1 tbsp fresh coriander, chopped
- 1 tbsp fresh mint, chopped
- freshly ground black pepper
- 1 small red onion, peeled and finely chopped
- 4 cherry tomatoes, halved
- 50g chickpeas (drained weight)
- 5 almonds
- 40g pomegranate seeds

Instructions:

Put the couscous in a mixing bowl and pour over the boiling water. Mix well, then cover with clingfilm and leave for 2-3 minutes until the water has been absorbed.

Place all of the other ingredients into a bowl and add the couscous. Mix together well, but be careful to not crush the tomatoes. Serve straight away or store in the fridge for up to 24 hours.

Simple Minestrone Soup

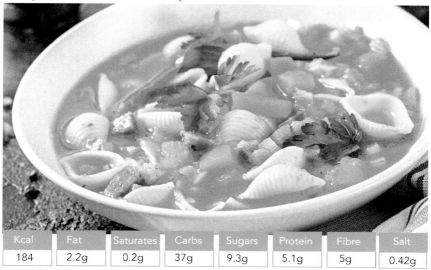

Kcal	Fat	Saturates	Carbs	Sugars	Protein	Fibre	Salt
184	2.2g	0.2g	37g	9.3g	5.1g	5g	0.42g

Serves: 2   **Prep time:** 5 minutes   **Cooking time:** 20 minutes

Ingredients:
- 1 celery stick, wiped and sliced
- 1 small carrot, peeled and diced
- 130g raw sweet potatoes, peeled and cut into 1cm cubes
- 50g pasta shells, dry weight
- 2 tsps tomato puree
- 500ml vegetable stock
- Rapeseed oil spray
- 1 shallot or small onion, peeled and finely diced
- ½ tsps Italian dried herbs
- salt and freshly ground black pepper
- fresh red chilli, for garnish (optional)
- fresh parsley, for garnish (optional)

Instructions:

Heat a medium-sized non-stick saucepan and add a couple of sprays of the rapeseed oil. Add the celery, sweet potato, diced shallot (or onion if using) and the diced carrot to the pan and gently fry for 3-4minutes.

Add the stock, herbs and tomato puree and bring to the boil then add the pasta shells. Cook for 10-12 minutes, or until the pasta is cooked to your liking.

Season to taste with the salt and a little black pepper.

Serve in warmed soup bowls topped with the fresh parsley and chilli if using.

Leftover Chicken Noodle Soup

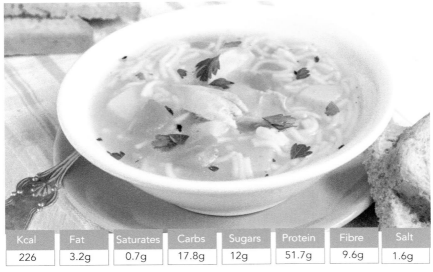

Kcal	Fat	Saturates	Carbs	Sugars	Protein	Fibre	Salt
226	3.2g	0.7g	17.8g	12g	51.7g	9.6g	1.6g

Serves: 1   **Prep time:** 5 minutes   **Cooking time:** 15 minutes

Ingredients:
- 100g cooked, leftover chicken, diced
- 250ml chicken stock
- 50g cooked, leftover potatoes, diced
- 50g cooked, leftover carrots
- 10g spaghetti, dry weight
- freshly ground black pepper
- fresh parsley, for garnish (optional)

Instructions:
Place the stock into a saucepan and bring to the boil. Break the spaghetti pasta into 2cm lengths and add to the boiling stock. Reduce the heat slightly and cook for 10 mins.

Add the diced chicken, potatoes and carrots to the stock and pasta. Reduce the heat to a gentle simmer and cook for a further 4-5 minutes.

Season with a little freshly ground black pepper and fresh parsley (if using) and serve straight away.

Super Easy Broccoli Soup

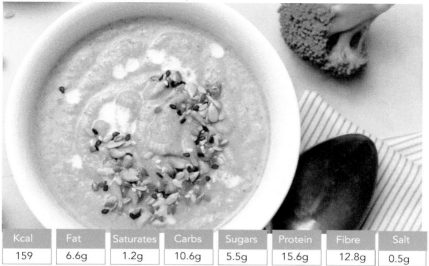

Kcal	Fat	Saturates	Carbs	Sugars	Protein	Fibre	Salt
159	6.6g	1.2g	10.6g	5.5g	15.6g	12.8g	0.5g

Serves: 1   **Prep time:** 5 minutes   **Cooking time:** 15 minutes

Ingredients:

- 300g frozen broccoli florets
- 175ml vegetable stock
- 1 tsp mixed seeds
- freshly ground black pepper
- 1 tsp yoghurt, for decoration, optional

Instructions:

Place the frozen broccoli in a small saucepan with the vegetable stock. Gently bring to the boil then reduce the heat slightly and cook for a further 10 minutes.

Remove the broccoli from the heat, season with a little black pepper and carefully transfer to a blender. Blitz until smooth.

Serve in a warmed soup bowl with the mixed seeds sprinkled over the top and a little yogurt (optional)

Tzatziki Style Crispbreads

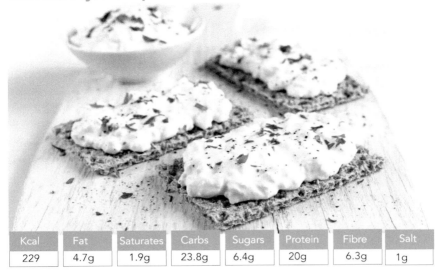

Kcal	Fat	Saturates	Carbs	Sugars	Protein	Fibre	Salt
229	4.7g	1.9g	23.8g	6.4g	20g	6.3g	1g

Serves: 1   **Prep time:** 5 minutes

Ingredients:
- 5 fresh mint leaves, chopped
- freshly ground black pepper
- 1 pinch garlic salt
- 150g low-fat natural cottage cheese
- 3 mulitgrain rye crispbreads, such as Ryvita

Instructions:
Place the cottage cheese in a small bowl and add the garlic salt, stir gently to combine.

Divide the cottage cheese mixture between the 3 crispbreads evenly. Sprinkle with a little freshly ground black pepper and top with the chopped mint. Serve straight away.

Tuna Salad Lettuce Wraps

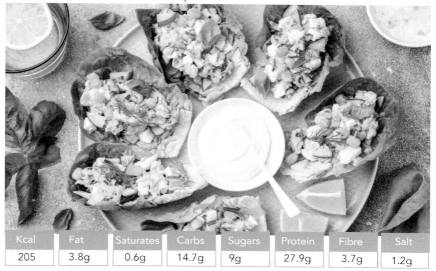

Kcal	Fat	Saturates	Carbs	Sugars	Protein	Fibre	Salt
205	3.8g	0.6g	14.7g	9g	27.9g	3.7g	1.2g

Serves: 1   **Prep time:** 5 minutes

Ingredients:

- 100g tuna chunks in brine, drained weight
- 6 baby gem lettuce leaves
- 50g sweetcorn
- 1 tbsp extra light mayonaise
- 2cm piece cucumber, diced
- ½ small red onion, peeled and finely diced
- 3 radishes, diced
- zest and juice of 1 small lemon

Instructions:

Place all of the ingredients except the lettuce leaves into a bowl and gently mix.

Divide the mixture equally between the 6 lettuce leaves and serve straight away with a little extra mayonnaise and basil leaves (optional)

Pearl Couscous Salad

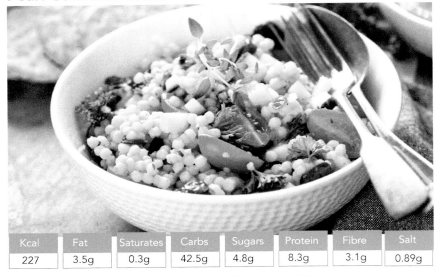

Kcal	Fat	Saturates	Carbs	Sugars	Protein	Fibre	Salt
227	3.5g	0.3g	42.5g	4.8g	8.3g	3.1g	0.89g

Serves: 1   **Prep time:** 5 minutes   **Cooking time:** 10 minutes

Ingredients:
- 50g pearl couscous
- salt and freshly ground black pepper
- Rapeseed oil spray
- 50g cucumber, diced
- ½ tsps dried mixed herbs
- 6 cherry tomatoes, quartered
- small handful fresh parsley, roughly chopped
- 10g dried cranberries, optional
- zest and juice of 1 lime
- 1 vegetable stock cube

Instructions:

Add a couple of sprays of the oil into a saucepan and heat. Add the couscous and gently fry for a couple of minutes until the couscous smells toasted, add the dried cranberries if using then cover with water and add the stock cube. Bring to the boil and simmer for 6-8 minutes, or until the couscous is just tender.

Using a sieve, drain the couscous and transfer to a bowl. Stir in the remaining ingredients. Season with a little salt and pepper.

Serve hot or cold.

Chickpeas and Mushrooms with Garlic

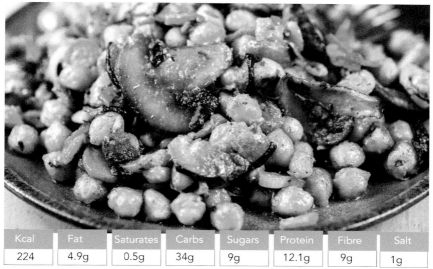

Kcal	Fat	Saturates	Carbs	Sugars	Protein	Fibre	Salt
224	4.9g	0.5g	34g	9g	12.1g	9g	1g

Serves: 1   **Prep time:** 5 minutes   **Cooking time:** 15 minutes

Ingredients:
- fresh parsley, chopped for serving (optional)
- 1 baby carrot, peeled and finely sliced
- salt and freshly ground black pepper, to season
- 100g chestnut mushrooms, cleaned and sliced
- 1x210g can of chickpeas, drained and rinsed
- 1 baby courgette, top and tailed, and thinly sliced
- Rapeseed oil spray
- 1 garlic clove, peeled and finely sliced
- 1 shallot, peeled and finely diced

Instructions:

Pre-heat a frying pan and add a couple of sprays of the rapeseed oil. Add the shallot and garlic and cook gently for 2-3 minutes.

Add the mushrooms, carrot and courgette and 1tbsp of water to the frying pan and cook for a further 4-6 minutes until they start to soften - if they become a little dry add a little more water.

Add the chickpeas and a little more water - about 1tbsp and cook for a further 3-4 minutes. Season with the salt and pepper and serve straight away garnished with the fresh parsley, or leave to cool and eat cold - this will keep in the fridge overnight.

Chunky Bean Soup

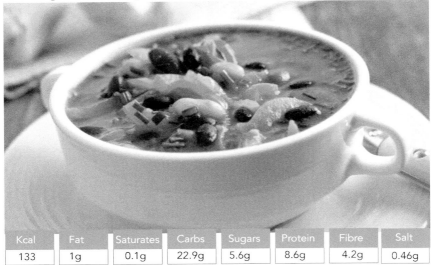

Kcal	Fat	Saturates	Carbs	Sugars	Protein	Fibre	Salt
133	1g	0.1g	22.9g	5.6g	8.6g	4.2g	0.46g

Serves: 4   **Prep time:** 10 minutes   **Cooking time:** 35 minutes

Ingredients:
- 1x200g tin of haricot beans, drained and rinsed
- 1x200g tin of flageolet beans, drained and rinsed
- 1x200g tin of kidney beans, drained and rinsed
- fresh chives, chopped for serving (optional)
- 200g tomato passata
- 0.8 litres Lactose and gluten free vegetable stock
- 1 red pepper and 1 yellow pepper, deseeded and diced
- salt and black pepper
- 1 medium onion, chopped
- 1 courgette, diced
- 2 tsps oregano or thyme, freshly chopped

Instructions:
Preheat a non-stick wok or frying pan. Dry-fry the onion and peppers for 4-5 minutes. Transfer to a large saucepan adding the remaining ingredients. Simmer gently for 30 minutes.

Allow to cool then divide into smaller containers. Seal and freeze. Reheat by bringing up to the boil and simmer for 10 minutes. Season to taste with salt and pepper and sprinkle over the chives if using.

TIP
A wholesome hearty lunch full of flavour. Made in large batches it will keep for up to five days in the refrigerator.

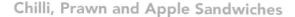

Chilli, Prawn and Apple Sandwiches

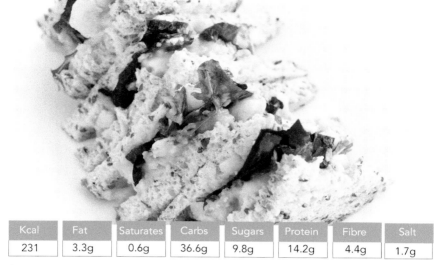

Kcal	Fat	Saturates	Carbs	Sugars	Protein	Fibre	Salt
231	3.3g	0.6g	36.6g	9.8g	14.2g	4.4g	1.7g

Serves: 2   **Prep time:** 10 minutes
Ingredients:
- 4 slices seedy bread
- 2 tbsps low-fat mayonnaise
- 2 tsps sweet chilli sauce
- 1 tsp lemon juice
- black pepper, freshly ground
- 100g cooked and peeled prawns
- 1 small eating apple, peeled, cored and grated
- salad leaves

Instructions:
Mix together the prawns, mayonnaise, chilli sauce, grated apple and lemon juice.

Spread the mixture on two slices of bread and top with salad leaves. Season with black pepper, and top with the two remaining slices of bread.

Cut into triangles and cover with food wrap until ready to serve.

Fried Egg with Spinach and Tomatoes

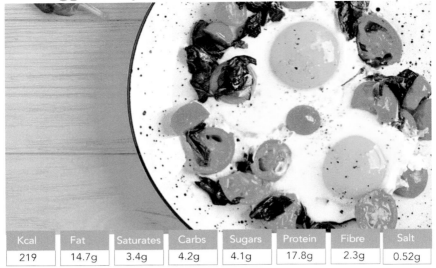

Kcal	Fat	Saturates	Carbs	Sugars	Protein	Fibre	Salt
219	14.7g	3.4g	4.2g	4.1g	17.8g	2.3g	0.52g

Serves: 1   **Prep time:** 5 minutes   **Cooking time:** 10 minutes

Ingredients:
- 2 medium sized eggs
- 10 cherry tomatoes, halved
- 50g baby spinach
- Rapeseed oil spray
- freshly ground black pepper

Instructions:
Heat a medium-sized non-stick frying pan and spray lightly with the rapeseed oil. Add the cherry tomatoes and gently fry for 2-3 minutes.

Add the baby spinach to the pan and stir.

Make a space in the middle of the frying pan add another couple of sprays of the rapeseed oil and carefully break the eggs into the center.

Reduce the heat slightly and cover the frying pan with a piece of foil (shiny side down) and allow the eggs to cook for 5 minutes.

Remove the foil, and transfer the eggs, spinach and tomatoes to a warmed plate. Season with the black pepper and serve.

Chicken and Watercress Salad

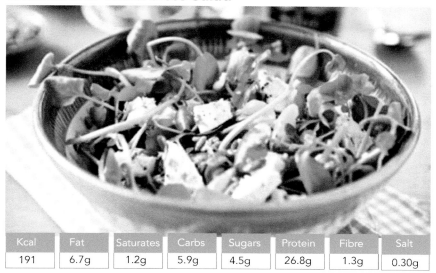

Kcal	Fat	Saturates	Carbs	Sugars	Protein	Fibre	Salt
191	6.7g	1.2g	5.9g	4.5g	26.8g	1.3g	0.30g

Serves: 1   **Prep time:** 10 minutes   **Cooking time:** 10 minutes

Ingredients:
- ½ tsps Agave syrup
- 40g fresh watercress
- 25g pickled Guindilla chillies
- 60g cooked chicken, cold and cut into strips
- 1 tbsp Fage Total 0% Greek Yogurt
- ½ tsps gluten free grain mustard
- 1 ½ tsps mixed (pumpkin, sesame) seeds
- 1 tsp lemon juice

Instructions:

Place the seeds on a non-stick baking tray and toast under a hot grill, then allow to cool.

Wash and drain the watercress and place in a serving bowl. Scatter over the chicken slices.

Mix together the dressing ingredients in a small bowl and drizzle over.

Top with chillies and the toasted seeds.

Puy Lentil and Pearl Couscous Vegetable Salad

Kcal	Fat	Saturates	Carbs	Sugars	Protein	Fibre	Salt
201	2.3g	0.4g	34.2g	11g	12g	9.7g	0.78g

Serves: 2   **Prep time:** 10 minutes   **Cooking time:** 50 minutes

Ingredients:
- 1x300g aubergine
- 75g Puy lentils, dry weight
- 25g Pearl couscous, dry weight
- 500ml vegetable stock
- 1x150g red peppers, de-seeded and diced
- 8 cherry tomatoes, cut into quarters
- 1 celery stick, finely diced
- ½ tsps cumin seeds
- 1 tsp parsley, finely chopped
- 1 tbsp of fresh mint, finely chopped
- 1 ½ tbsps white wine vinegar
- ½ tsps Dijon mustard
- balsamic vinegar
- salt and freshly ground black pepper

Instructions:
Pre-heat the oven to 200C, 400F, gas mark 6. Place the aubergine on a baking tray and cook for 40 minutes, then remove from the oven and allow to cool.

Whilst the aubergine is baking add the stock to a medium-sized saucepan and bring to the boil. Add the puy lentils and reduce the heat slightly and cook for 20 minutes.

Once the lentils are cooked remove from the heat and add the pearl couscous to the saucepan, stir gently and then set aside to cool.

Remove the stalk from the cooked aubergine and cut the flesh into 1cm cubes and transfer to a large mixing bowl with the chopped pepper, celery, tomatoes and the chopped fresh mint and parsley.

In a small bowl mix together the dijon mustard, white wine vinegar and add some freshly ground black pepper.

Once the pearl couscous has become soft (but not mushy texture) drain the lentil/couscous mixture discarding any remaining liquid. Transfer the lentils and couscous to the bowl with the vegetables and pour over the dressing. Stir gently to combine. Season with a little salt if required. Transfer to the fridge for 30 minutes to allow the flavours to develop (or overnight). Serve drizzled with a little balsamic dressing.

Tuna Pate

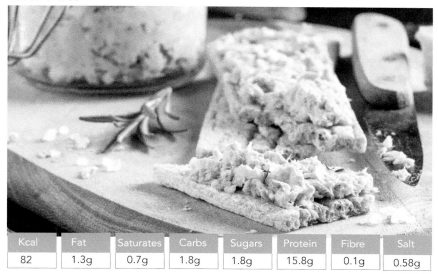

Kcal	Fat	Saturates	Carbs	Sugars	Protein	Fibre	Salt
82	1.3g	0.7g	1.8g	1.8g	15.8g	0.1g	0.58g

Serves: 1   **Prep time:** 5 minutes

Ingredients:
- juice from 1 lime
- black pepper
- 60g extra light soft cheese
- 100g tuna in brine, drained weight

Instructions:
Place all of the ingredients into a bowl and mash together using a fork. Adjust the seasoning with a little more black pepper if required. Store in the fridge for up to two days.

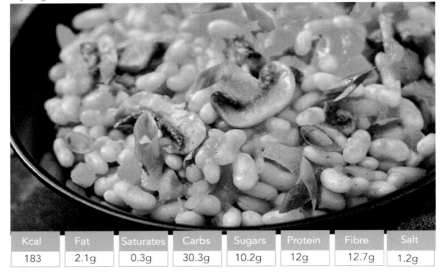

Kcal	Fat	Saturates	Carbs	Sugars	Protein	Fibre	Salt
183	2.1g	0.3g	30.3g	10.2g	12g	12.7g	1.2g

Serves: 2   **Prep time:** 5 minutes   **Cooking time:** 15 minutes

Ingredients:
- 1x415g can of no-added sugar baked beans
- 100g mushrooms, cleaned and sliced
- 2 spring onions, cleaned, root removed and sliced
- 1 small red pepper, deseeded and diced
- ½ tsps chilli powder
- Rapeseed oil spray

Instructions:
Preheat a small frying pan and add a couple of sprays of the rapeseed oil. Add the spring onion, diced pepper and sliced mushrooms and cook for 5-6 minutes.

Add the chilli powder and stir to combine then add the baked beans, reduce the heat to a simmer and cook for a further 5 minutes. Serve hot

TIP
These are great on toast or served with a jacket potato.

Melon, Prosciutto and Olive Salad

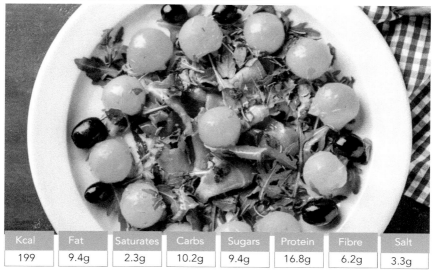

Kcal	Fat	Saturates	Carbs	Sugars	Protein	Fibre	Salt
199	9.4g	2.3g	10.2g	9.4g	16.8g	6.2g	3.3g

Serves: 1   **Prep time:** 10 minutes

Ingredients:
- 2 slices (42g) Prosciutto ham
- 230g cantaloup melon, cut into pieces or balls
- 6 black olives
- 100g rocket leaves or
- 1 tbsp fat free french dressing

Instructions:

Place the rocket or salad leaves in a bowl and pour over the salad dressing. Gently toss until evenly coated in the dressing.

Place the Proscuitto ham in the center of a serving plate and scatter the Rocket or salad leaves around the side.

Top with the melon pieces and garnish with the black olives. Serve straight away.

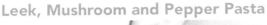

Leek, Mushroom and Pepper Pasta

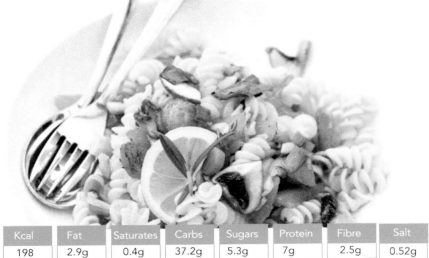

Kcal	Fat	Saturates	Carbs	Sugars	Protein	Fibre	Salt
198	2.9g	0.4g	37.2g	5.3g	7g	2.5g	0.52g

Serves: 4   **Prep time:** 10 minutes   **Cooking time:** 20 minutes

Ingredients:
- 180g dry pasta shapes
- 200g leeks, sliced
- 2 tbsps basil leaf, chopped for garnish
- salt and freshly ground black pepper
- 2 tsps basil pesto
- 1 vegetable stock cube
- 200g chestnut mushrooms, sliced
- 1 yellow pepper, diced
- 3 spring onions, cleaned and sliced
- 1 long red pepper, diced

Instructions:
Heat a non-stick pan, and dry-fry the vegetables for 10 minutes until soft. Season with salt and pepper.

Cook the pasta in a large pan of boiling water containing the stock cube.

Drain the pasta thoroughly, then tip it back into the pan. Add the vegetables and pesto, mixing well. Divide between 4 warmed serving plates and garnish with the fresh basil. Serve with a large mixed salad.

TIP
Add a pinch of dried chilli flakes to spice up the sauce.

Butter Bean Soup

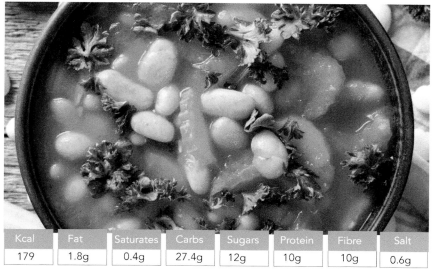

Kcal	Fat	Saturates	Carbs	Sugars	Protein	Fibre	Salt
179	1.8g	0.4g	27.4g	12g	10g	10g	0.6g

Serves: 2   **Prep time:** 5 minutes   **Cooking time:** 25 minutes

Ingredients:
- 1x400g tin of butter beans, drained
- 300g tomato passata
- 1 celery stick, sliced
- 1 small carrot, peeled and sliced
- 1 small onion, peeled and finely diced
- 1 gluten and lactose free vegetable stock cube, crumbled
- salt and freshly ground black pepper
- Rapeseed oil spray
- fresh parsley, for garnish (optional)

Instructions:

Heat a medium-sized saucepan and add a couple of sprays of the rapeseed oil and add the onion, celery, sliced carrots and garlic and cook for 3-4 minutes.

Add the tomato passata, vegetable stock cube and 100ml of warm water to the saucepan and bring to the boil.

Once the liquid has come to the boil add the drained butter beans, a little salt and black pepper, reduce the heat slightly to a strong simmer and cook for further 20 minutes.

Serve the soup in warmed bowls topped with a little fresh parsley (optional).

Fish Soup

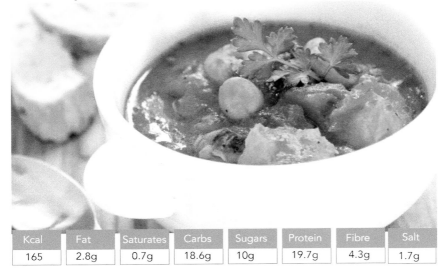

Kcal	Fat	Saturates	Carbs	Sugars	Protein	Fibre	Salt
165	2.8g	0.7g	18.6g	10g	19.7g	4.3g	1.7g

Serves: 1   **Prep time:** 5 minutes   **Cooking time:** 20 minutes

Ingredients:
- 2 spring onions, cleaned, root removed and sliced
- 200g tomato passata
- 120ml chicken stock
- 120g Frozen mixed fish and seafood, defrosted and any fish cut into small chunks
- 1 tsp fresh parsley, chopped
- ½ tsps smoked paprika
- black pepper
- Rapeseed oil spray

Instructions:

Heat a saucepan over a medium heat and add a couple sprays of the rapeseed oil. Add the spring onion, garlic paste and paprika and cook for 2-3 mins stirring occasionally, then pour in the tomato passata and chicken stock. Season with a little black pepper. Bring to the boil, then reduce to a simmer for 6-7 mins.

Add the fish and seafood mix and continue cooking for 5-6 mins, stir in the parsley.

Pour the soup into a warmed bowl and serve straight away.

Edamame and Mushroom Salad

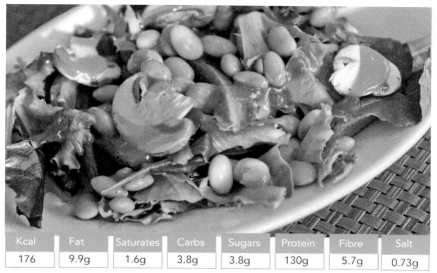

Kcal	Fat	Saturates	Carbs	Sugars	Protein	Fibre	Salt
176	9.9g	1.6g	3.8g	3.8g	130g	5.7g	0.73g

Serves: 1   **Prep time:** 5 minutes

Ingredients:
- 1 tbsp Blue Dragon Sweet Chilli Sauce
- 2 large handfuls mixed salad leaves
- 60g chestnut mushrooms, cleaned and sliced
- 80g ready to eat Edamame beans

Instructions:
Place the salad leaves on a plate and top with the ready to eat edamame beans and sliced mushrooms. Drizzle over the sweet chilli sauce and serve straight away

Indian Style Roasted Cauliflower Steak

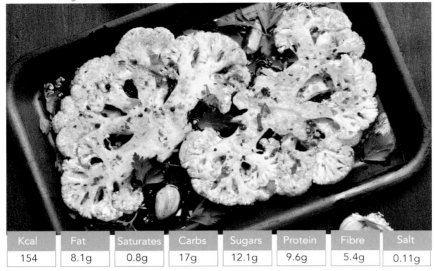

Kcal	Fat	Saturates	Carbs	Sugars	Protein	Fibre	Salt
154	8.1g	0.8g	17g	12.1g	9.6g	5.4g	0.11g

Serves: 1 **Prep time:** 5 minutes **Cooking time:** 20 minutes

Ingredients:
- 2 large slices of cauliflower, cut approx. 1 ½cm thick
- 1 clove of garlic, peeled and crushed
- 1 tsp rapeseed oil
- 1 tsp golden syrup
- ½ tsps turmeric
- ¼ tsps fennel seed
- ¼ tsps mustard seed
- ¼ tsps ground cumin

Instructions:
Preheat the oven to 200C, Gas Mark 6, 400F In a small bowl mix together the turmeric, rapeseed oil, golden syrup, mustard seeds, fennel seeds and ground cumin to form a paste.

Brush both sides of the cauliflower slices with the spicy paste mix and lay on a non-stick baking tray. Lay the crushed garlic in between the cauliflower slices.

When cooked discard the garlic and serve immediately – sprinkle over some fresh herbs (optional).

Vegetarian Stuffed Peppers

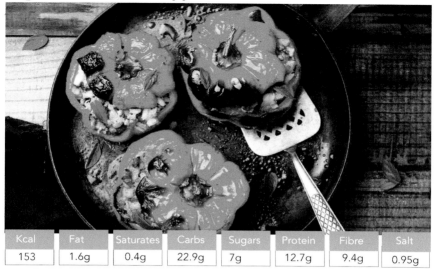

Kcal	Fat	Saturates	Carbs	Sugars	Protein	Fibre	Salt
153	1.6g	0.4g	22.9g	7g	12.7g	9.4g	0.95g

Serves: 3   **Prep time:** 10 minutes   **Cooking time:** 40 minutes

Ingredients:

- 55g basmati rice
- 200g Lactose and gluten free Quorn mince
- 3 large red peppers
- 1 medium red onion, finely chopped
- 1 garlic clove, peeled and finely chopped
- 100g button mushrooms, cleaned and finely chopped
- 1 tbsp fresh coriander, finely chopped
- 100ml vegetable stock

Instructions:

Preheat the oven to 180C.

Bring a small saucepan of water to the boil and add the basmati rice. Cook for 8-10 minutes, then drain.

Heat a large non-stick frying pan and cook the onions and garlic until just turning light brown. Add the chopped mushrooms, cooked rice, Quorn mince, tomato puree, coriander and vegetable stock, stir well and cook for 4-5 minutes.

Clean and carefully cut the tops off the peppers, and using a spoon remove the insides including the seeds.

Fill the peppers with the mince mixture, press in the mince filling in with a spoon and fill to the top. Put the 'lids' back on and place firmly in an ovenproof dish so that they stay upright.

Bake for 25 minutes.

Carpaccio of Beef

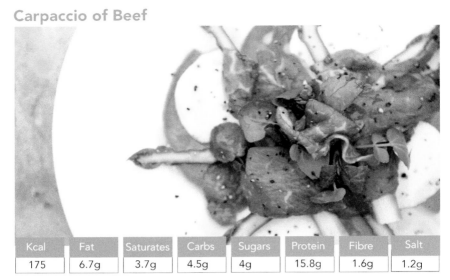

Kcal	Fat	Saturates	Carbs	Sugars	Protein	Fibre	Salt
175	6.7g	3.7g	4.5g	4g	15.8g	1.6g	1.2g

Serves: 4   **Prep time:** 12 hours

Ingredients:
- 200g lean beef fillet
- 1 tsp sea salt
- 2 garlic cloves, finely chopped
- 100ml fresh orange juice
- 80g reduced-fat mozzarella cheese
- chives, to serve
- 1 pinch black pepper, coarsely ground
- 200ml red wine

Instructions:

Trim any fat from the meat with a sharp knife and place in a small cereal bowl, so the marinade will cover it completely. Rub the meat with salt and black pepper to coat.

Sprinkle with garlic and combine the wine and orange juice before pouring over. Cover with food wrap and refrigerate overnight.

Snap the stems from the asparagus at the lowest point and blanch together in a pan of boiling water for 2-3 minutes until just cooked, then strain and rinse in cold water.

Slice the mozzarella and arrange on serving plates with the tomato slices and blanched asparagus. Remove the meat from the marinade and slice, using a sharp knife, placing the slices on to a chopping board.

Cover the board with 2 sheets of clear food wrap then roll into thin slices using a rolling pin. Using a palette knife, carefully lift the beef slices from the board and arrange on top of the salad plate.

Drizzle with some of the marinade and serve with fresh chives.

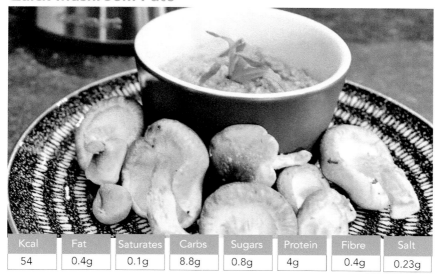

Kcal	Fat	Saturates	Carbs	Sugars	Protein	Fibre	Salt
54	0.4g	0.1g	8.8g	0.8g	4g	0.4g	0.23g

Serves: 2 **Prep time:** 5 minutes **Cooking time:** 10 minutes

Ingredients:

- 1 tbsp water
- 1 tsp dark soy sauce or gluten free soy sauce
- 100g canned haricot beans, drained
- 1 clove of garlic, peeled
- 100g mixed mushrooms, wiped clean, and sliced

Instructions:

Place the mushrooms, garlic and water into a small frying pan and cook for 3-4 minutes until the mushrooms and garlic have softened

Transfer the cooked mushrooms and garlic to a bowl with the drained haricot beans and soy sauce, and using a stick blender blend until smooth. (you can do this in a small food processor).

Place the pate mixture into a small non-metallic bowl and allow to cool. Then cover in clingfilm, chill in the fridge for 20 minutes and then serve.

Serve with crackers or bread.

TIP

This will keep for 2-3 days in the fridge

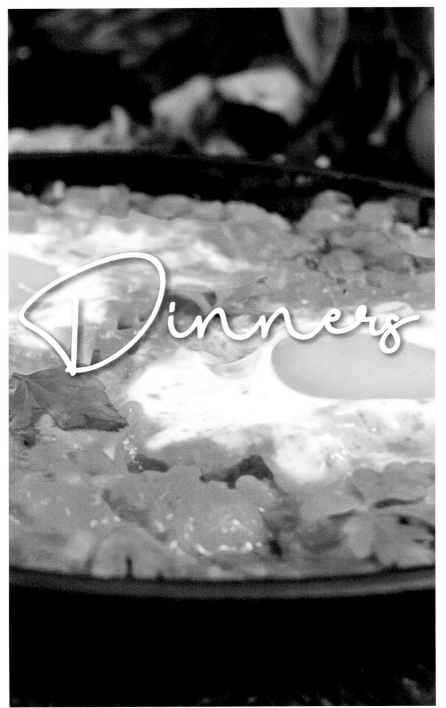

Dinners

Cheats Sausage Jambalaya

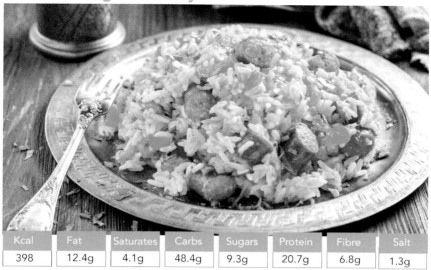

Kcal	Fat	Saturates	Carbs	Sugars	Protein	Fibre	Salt
398	12.4g	4.1g	48.4g	9.3g	20.7g	6.8g	1.3g

Serves: 2   **Prep time:** 5 minutes   **Cooking time:** 10 minutes

Ingredients:

- ¼ tsps chilli powder, optional
- 1x250g packet ready cooked Mexican style rice
- 1 small red pepper, de-seeded and diced
- 1 small onion, peeled and finely diced
- 3 reduced-fat pork sausages or plant-based sausages, each cut into 6 pieces
- freshly ground black pepper
- Rapeseed oil spray
- fresh parsley, to garnish, optional

Instructions:

Heat a frying pan and add a couple of sprays of rapeseed oil. Add the onion, red pepper and sausage pieces and cook for 4-5 minutes, stirring occasionally.

Add the Mexican style rice and chilli powder (if using) to the frying pan with 3 tablespoons of water and cook for a further 3-4 minutes, stirring occasionally.

Remove from the heat and serve straight away with a little fresh parsley.

Honey and Thyme Baked Salmon

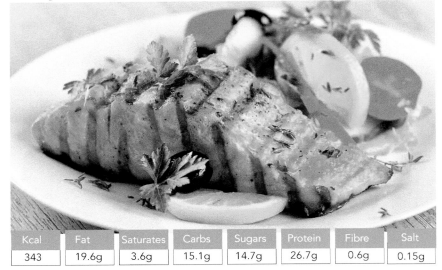

Kcal	Fat	Saturates	Carbs	Sugars	Protein	Fibre	Salt
343	19.6g	3.6g	15.1g	14.7g	26.7g	0.6g	0.15g

Serves: 2   **Prep time:** 15 minutes   **Cooking time:** 15 minutes

Ingredients:
- 2x130g salmon fillets
- juice of 1 lemon
- 2 tbsps honey
- 1 sprig of thyme
- parsley, to garnish, optional

Instructions:
Preheat the oven to 190C, Gas Mark 5, 375F

In a bowl mix together the lemon juice, honey and fresh thyme to make the marinade. Place the salmon fillets flesh side down into the marinade and leave for 10 minutes.

Remove the salmon from the marinade and place the fillets skin side down into an ovenproof dish and pour over the honey marinade. Cook for 12- 15 minutes until cooked to your liking.

Serve the salmon with the thyme sprig and fresh parsley sprinkled over the top. Serve hot or cold.

TIP
You can also cook this in a griddle pan or on the BBQ.

Quick Frozen Veg Pizza

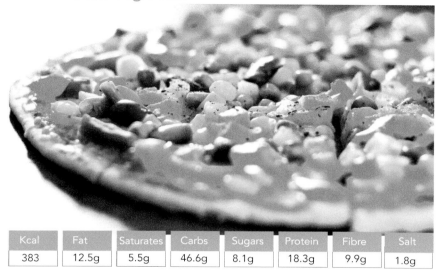

Kcal	Fat	Saturates	Carbs	Sugars	Protein	Fibre	Salt
383	12.5g	5.5g	46.6g	8.1g	18.3g	9.9g	1.8g

Serves: 1   **Prep time:** 5 minutes   **Cooking time:** 12 minutes

Ingredients:

- 25g reduced-fat mozzarella or vegan style cheddar cheese
- 3 black olives, sliced (optional)
- 160g frozen mixed vegetables, such as peas, sweetcorn, peppers etc
- ½ tsps Italian dried herbs
- 3 tsps tomato puree
- 1 wholewheat soft tortilla wrap

Instructions:

Pre-heat the oven to 200C, 400F, gas mark 6.

Place the soft tortilla wrap on a non-stick baking tray. Spread the tomato puree over the top and sprinkle with the dried mixed herbs.

Evenely coat with the frozen mixed vegetables and olives if using. Sprinkle over the grated cheese and bake in the oven for 12 minutes or until the cheese is bubbling.

Serve hot or cold.

TIP

Using vegan style cheese makes this recipe lactose free.

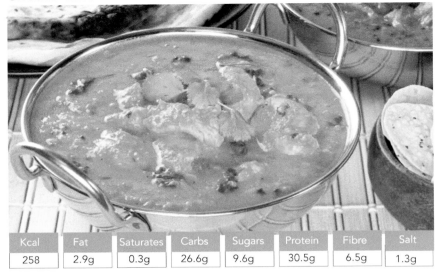

Kcal	Fat	Saturates	Carbs	Sugars	Protein	Fibre	Salt
258	2.9g	0.3g	26.6g	9.6g	30.5g	6.5g	1.3g

Serves: 2   **Prep time:** 5 minutes   **Cooking time:** 25 minutes

Ingredients:
- 1 large white onion, finely diced
- 1x400g lentil soup
- 200g raw skinless chicken breasts, chopped into cubes
- 1 red chilli, finely chopped
- 1 garlic clove, peeled and finely chopped
- 3 tsps garam masala
- 1x200g tin of chopped tomatoes
- 1 tbsp fresh coriander, chopped to serve
- oil spray

Instructions:
Heat a heavy based large saucepan and spray with the oil spray. Add the onion, garlic and chilli cook gently until softened.

Now add the chicken pieces and cook for a further 5 mins.

Add the garam masala, tomatoes and lentil soup to the chicken. Stir and reduce to a simmer.

Cook for a further 20 minutes until the sauce has thickened or transfer to a slowcooker and cook as per your slowcooker instructions - normally 2-3 hours on low.

Stir in the fresh coriander just before serving. Serve with basmati rice or a naan bread (calories for these are not included).

TIP
You can cook this in a slowcooker - allow 2-3 hours depending on your slow cooker instructions.

Smoked Cod with Rice and Red Peppers

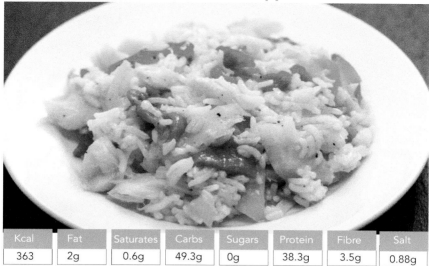

Kcal	Fat	Saturates	Carbs	Sugars	Protein	Fibre	Salt
363	2g	0.6g	49.3g	0g	38.3g	3.5g	0.88g

Serves: 1   **Prep time:** 5 minutes   **Cooking time:** 20 minutes

Ingredients:

- 180g smoked cod, bones removed
- 120g ready roasted red peppers, homemade or from a jar
- 55g basmati rice, dry weight
- 250ml semi-skimmed milk
- 1 bay leaf
- 4 peppercorns
- 1 vegetable stock cube
- freshly ground black pepper

Instructions:

Bring a pan of water to the boil and add the stock cube then the rice, bring back to the boil and reduce the heat slightly so the water is gently bubbling.

In a small frying pan add the bay leaf, pinch of salt, a few peppercorns and heat the milk until a gentle simmer. Add the cod and cook for 5-8 minutes.

Just before the rice is cooked add the pepper slices to the rice and cook for a further minute. Drain the rice and return to the pan but do not cook any further.

Gently remove the fish from the frying pan and discard the milk and herbs. Gently flake the fish into chunks and transfer to the rice and peppers. Stir very gently so not to mash up the cod flakes.

Transfer to a warmed bowl and season with a little salt and pepper.

Pan Fried Salmon on a Bed of Wilted Spinach, Mushrooms and Yoghurt

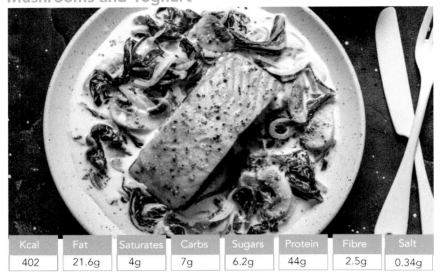

Kcal	Fat	Saturates	Carbs	Sugars	Protein	Fibre	Salt
402	21.6g	4g	7g	6.2g	44g	2.5g	0.34g

Serves: 1   **Prep time:** 5 minutes   **Cooking time:** 20 minutes

Ingredients:
- 100g low-fat Greek yoghurt
- 1x140g salmon fillet
- 1 shallot or small onion, peeled and finely sliced
- 80g chestnut mushrooms, sliced
- 80g baby spinach
- freshly ground black pepper
- Rapeseed oil spray

Instructions:
Season the salmon with some black pepper. Preheat a medium frying pan and add a couple of sprays of rapeseed oil and add the salmon skin side down. Add the sliced mushrooms and onions to the frying pan with the fish, stirring occasionally so they cook evenly.

After about 6-8 minutes turn the salmon over and continue to cook for a further 3-4 minutes or until the salmon is cooked to your liking. Remove the salmon from the pan and transfer to a warmed serving plate, leaving the mushrooms and onions in the frying pan.

Add the spinach to the mushroom and onions and cook for 1-2 minutes until the spinach has wilted. Reduce the heat and add the yoghurt stirring gently so that the yoghurt does not separate and mixes with the juices in the pan. Cook very gently for a further 1-2 minutes. Season with freshly ground black pepper and pour the mixture around the salmon.

Serve straight away.

Chinese Style Tempeh

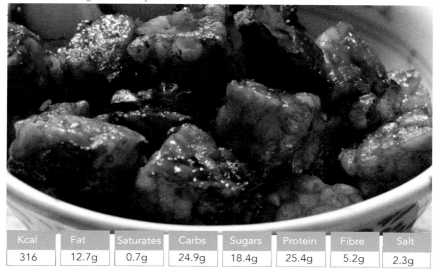

Kcal	Fat	Saturates	Carbs	Sugars	Protein	Fibre	Salt
316	12.7g	0.7g	24.9g	18.4g	25.4g	5.2g	2.3g

Serves: 1   **Prep time:** 5 minutes   **Cooking time:** 10 minutes

Ingredients:

- 120g Tempeh, cut into 1cm cubes
- 1 tbsp golden syrup
- 2 tsps dark soy sauce
- 1 tsp sesame oil
- ½ tsps Chinese five spice

Instructions:

Place the golden syrup, dark soy sauce, sesame oil and Chinese five-spice into a medium bowl and mix together.

Add the cubed Tempeh, and stir so that it is completely coated in the marinade.

Cover the bowl with clingfilm, and refrigerate for at least 1 hour (this can be done overnight if you prefer).

Heat a medium frying pan until hot, and the tempeh cubes and fry for 5-10 minutes until heated through and the syrup starts to caramelise, pour over any remaining marinade and serve straight away.

Great served with rice or noodles.

TIP

You can leave this to marinate overnight if you prefer.

Chicken and Chickpea Casserole

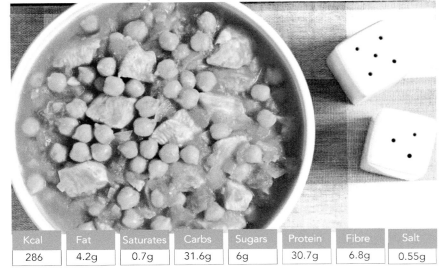

Kcal	Fat	Saturates	Carbs	Sugars	Protein	Fibre	Salt
286	4.2g	0.7g	31.6g	6g	30.7g	6.8g	0.55g

Serves: 4   **Prep time:** 5 minutes   **Cooking time:** 50 minutes

Ingredients:
- 2 tsps smoked paprika
- 300g skinless chicken breasts, cubed
- 1 red onion, finely diced
- 1 green pepper, cored, de-seeded and chopped
- 2 turkey rashers, sliced into strips
- 2 garlic cloves
- 200g sweet potatoes, peeled and cubed into cm pieces
- 2 carrots, peeled and diced
- 50g red lentils (dry weight)
- 1x400g tin of chickpeas, drained
- oil spray
- 750ml chicken stock

Instructions:
Heat a heavy deep based frying pan and spray with the oil spray. Gently cook the onion, garlic and green pepper until softened.

Add the chicken and turkey and cook for a further 5 minutes, stirring occasionally.

Add the remaining ingredients, reduce the heat to a simmer and cook for a further 40 minutes.

Serve in large warmed bowls.

Rich Sausage and Mushroom Casserole

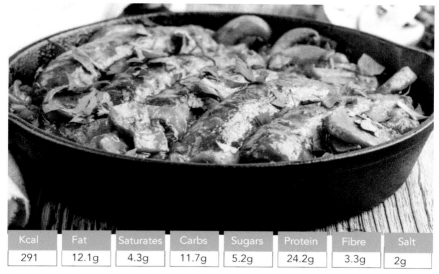

Kcal	Fat	Saturates	Carbs	Sugars	Protein	Fibre	Salt
291	12.1g	4.3g	11.7g	5.2g	24.2g	3.3g	2g

Serves: 3   **Prep time:** 5 minutes   **Cooking time:** 45 minutes

Ingredients:
- 6 reduced-fat pork sausages
- 200g tomato passata
- 150g chestnut mushrooms, wiped and sliced
- 1 red onion, peeled and diced
- 150ml full bodied red wine, such as Malbec
- 150ml beef stock
- 1 tsp smoked paprika
- 1 clove of garlic, peeled and diced
- 1 tsp fresh thyme
- salt and freshly ground black pepper
- Rapeseed oil spray

Instructions:
Heat a large heavy-based pan and add a couple of sprays of rapeseed oil and add the diced onion and garlic and cook gently for 3-4 minutes.

Add the sausages to the pan and cook for 4-6 minutes until browned

Add the sliced mushrooms, smoked paprika and red wine, stir gently then add the tomato passata and fresh thyme.

Stir in the beef stock and reduce the heat to a simmer. Cook for 30-35 minutes.

Season with a little salt and black pepper, then sprinkle over a little fresh parsley and serve straight away.

Beef and Black Pudding Kofta Kebabs

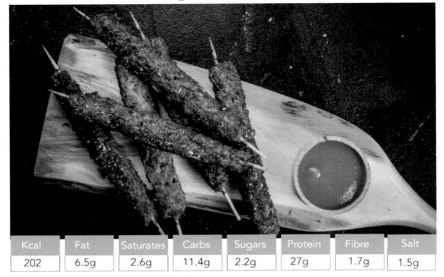

Kcal	Fat	Saturates	Carbs	Sugars	Protein	Fibre	Salt
202	6.5g	2.6g	11.4g	2.2g	27g	1.7g	1.5g

Serves: 2   **Prep time:** 40 minutes   **Cooking time:** 10 minutes

Ingredients:
- 200g lean beef mince
- 100g black pudding
- 1 tsp ground cumin
- ½ tsps paprika
- 1 pinch cayenne pepper
- 1 pinch salt and black pepper

Instructions:
Place the black pudding into a food processor and blitz until it resembles a breadcrumb texture.

Transfer the black pudding crumb to a mixing bowl and add the other ingredients. Mix all of the ingredients together, cover in clingfilm and let it rest for 30 minutes or overnight in the fridge.

Divide the mixture into four equal quantities and shape them into sausage shapes. Slide a skewer up through the middle.

Pre-heat a griddle pan or grill to hot. Cook the kebabs on one side for 5 minutes then carefully turn over and cook for a further 4 minutes. Serve straight away.

TIP
These are great on a BBQ.

Carrot Chips

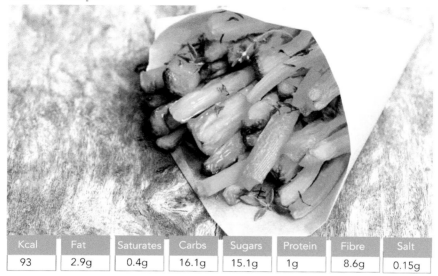

Kcal	Fat	Saturates	Carbs	Sugars	Protein	Fibre	Salt
93	2.9g	0.4g	16.1g	15.1g	1g	8.6g	0.15g

Serves: 1   **Prep time:** 5 minutes   **Cooking time:** 20 minutes

Ingredients:
- 240g carrots, peeled and cut into chips
- Rapeseed oil spray

Instructions:

Preheat the oven to 200C, 400F, gas mark 6

Line a baking tray with baking parchment. Spread the carrot batons over the baking tray and spray lightly with the rapeseed oil.

Bake for 12 minutes then turn the carrots over, return to the oven for another 8 minutes or until they start to caramelise. Best served hot

TIP

These are a great alternative to potato chips.

Kcal	Fat	Saturates	Carbs	Sugars	Protein	Fibre	Salt
348	10.3g	4g	33g	8.7g	31.4g	4.7g	0.98g

Serves: 2   **Prep time:** 5 minutes   **Cooking time:** 12 minutes

Ingredients:
- 2 tbsps tomato puree
- 120g cooked chicken, sliced
- 2 mini naan breads
- 45g reduced-fat Cheddar cheese, grated
- 1 small red pepper, de-seeded and cut into thin strips
- ½ red onion, peeled and thinly sliced
- 1 tomato, de-seeded and cut into thin strips
- 1 tsp Italian dried herbs
- 1 spring onion, slicedy

Instructions:
Pre-heat the oven to 185C.

Evenly spread the tomato puree over the naan breads then place them on to a baking tray. Lay the slices of tomato over the top and sprinkle with the herbs.

Add the chopped chicken, and red peppers, then sprinkle over the cheese. Top with the sliced onion and bake in the oven for 10-12 minutes until cooked.

Garnish with the chopped spring onion (optional) Serve hot or cold.

Stuffed Aubergine with Red Lentils

Kcal	Fat	Saturates	Carbs	Sugars	Protein	Fibre	Salt
378	7.3g	3.2g	56.9g	27g	25.4g	5.7g	1.7g

Serves: 1 **Prep time:** 10 minutes **Cooking time:** 45 minutes

Ingredients:
- 40g reduced fat feta cheese or vegan style feta cheese, crumbled
- 150g tomato passata
- 40g split red lentils
- 1 tbsp sultanas
- ¼ tsps dried mixed herbs
- ¼ tsps ground cinnamon
- ½ tsps smoked paprika
- 1 small carrot, peeled and grated
- 50g chestnut mushrooms, cleaned and diced
- 2 spring onions, cleaned, root removed and chopped
- 1 garlic clove, peeled and finely chopped
- 1 medium aubergine, cut in half, length ways

Instructions:

Bring a large pan of water to the boil. Place the aubergine halves into the boiling water and allow to cook for 3-4 minutes. Carefully remove from the water and allow to drain and cool for a couple of minutes. Carefully scoop out the cooked flesh of the aubergine making sure you don't pierce the skins. Roughly chop the flesh and set aside.

Heat a frying pan, and add a couple of sprays of rapeseed oil and the garlic and the spring onions and cook for 1-2 minutes, Add the chopped aubergine flesh, chopped mushrooms and grated carrot. Stir gently and cook for another minute.

Add the ground cinnamon, smoked paprika, dried mixed herbs, sultanas and split red lentils and the crush tomatoes. Stir occasionally and cook for 10 -15 minutes until the lentils have softened.

Preheat the oven to 190C, gas mark 5. Place the aubergine shells on a non-stick baking tray and divide the stuffing mixture equally between the two halves. Sprinkle over the crumble feta style cheese and bake in the oven for 10-15 minutes.

Serve straight away.

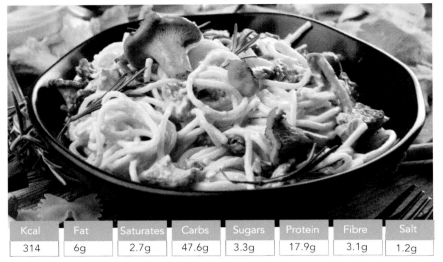

Kcal	Fat	Saturates	Carbs	Sugars	Protein	Fibre	Salt
314	6g	2.7g	47.6g	3.3g	17.9g	3.1g	1.2g

Serves: 2   **Prep time:** 5 minutes   **Cooking time:** 20 minutes

Ingredients:
- 260g mixed fresh mushrooms, cleaned and cut in half
- 120g spaghetti, dry weight
- 2 tsps Marmite or Vegemite
- 20g Parmesan or Pecorino cheese, finely grated
- 60g low-fat cream cheese
- 1 clove of garlic, peeled and finely diced
- freshly ground black pepper
- Rapeseed oil spray
- a couple of sprigs of fresh rosemary, for garnish (optional)

Instructions:
Bring a large pan of water to the boil. Add the spaghetti and cook.

Whilst the spaghetti is cooking, heat a frying pan and add a couple of sprays of the rapeseed oil and add the garlic and gently cook until softened.

Add the mixed mushrooms to the frying pan with the garlic and cook for 4-5 minutes until they start to soften, then stir in the Marmite and cream cheese and season with a little black pepper.

Add 3 tablespoons of the hot pasta water to the frying pan the make a sauce a little thinner and stir to ensure there are no lumps. Stir in the finely grated Parmesan and reduce the heat to low. (If the sauce feels a bit thick, add another tablespoon of the hot pasta water).

Drain the spaghetti and add the to mushrooms and Marmite sauce, stir gently to combine and serve in warmed pasta bowls with a little fresh Rosemary sprinkled over the top (optional).

Griddled Chicken with Wedges and Roasted Tomatoes

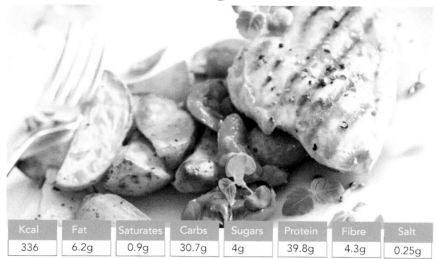

Kcal	Fat	Saturates	Carbs	Sugars	Protein	Fibre	Salt
336	6.2g	0.9g	30.7g	4g	39.8g	4.3g	0.25g

Serves: 1   **Prep time:** 5 minutes   **Cooking time:** 25 minutes

Ingredients:
- 1x150g skinless chicken breast
- 1x150g potato, skin on, cut into 8 wedges
- 8 cherry tomatoes, stalks removed
- Rapeseed oil spray
- freshly ground black pepper

Instructions:
Pre-heat the oven to 200C, 400F, Gas mark 6.

Place the potato wedges on a non-stick baking tray leaving a space in the middle for the tomatoes (which will be added later on). Spray the wedges with a little rapeseed oil spray and put in the oven.

Place the chicken fillet onto a chopping board, using a rolling pin gently bash the chicken breast to flatten it out slightly. Heat a griddle pan or frying pan and add a couple of sprays of the rapeseed oil. Place the chicken in the griddle pan or frying pan and cook for 10-12 minutes on each side, or until cooked.

Whilst the chicken is cooking on the first side, carefully remove the wedges from the oven and turn over. Add the tomatoes to the tray and return to the oven until the wedges are golden brown and the tomatoes are soft.

Once the chicken is cooked, rest for a couple of minutes. Season with a little freshly ground black pepper and serve with the potatoes and roasted tomatoes.

Quick Bacon Spaghetti Carbonara

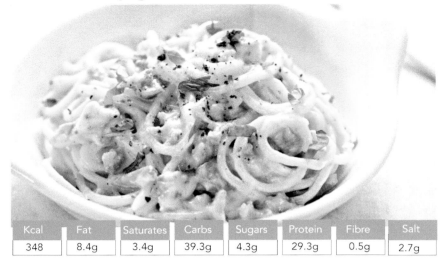

Kcal	Fat	Saturates	Carbs	Sugars	Protein	Fibre	Salt
348	8.4g	3.4g	39.3g	4.3g	29.3g	0.5g	2.7g

Serves: 1   **Prep time:** 5 minutes   **Cooking time:** 15 minutes

Ingredients:
- freshly ground black pepper
- 60g Extra Light low fat cream cheese
- 50g spaghetti or gluten free spaghetti, dry weight
- 3 rashers lean back bacon

Instructions:
Cook the spaghetti in boiling water for 10 minutes.

While the spaghetti is cooking, Dry fry bacon and then cut the bacon into small strips.

Drain the spaghetti and add the bacon, and cream cheese. Return to a low heat and gently stir until the cheese has melted and has coated the pasta and bacon.

Season with freshly ground black pepper Serve in a warm pasta bowl.

Cod on a Bed of Smoky Butter Beans

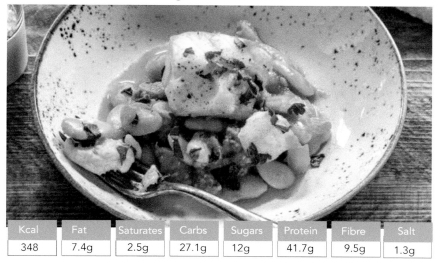

Kcal	Fat	Saturates	Carbs	Sugars	Protein	Fibre	Salt
348	7.4g	2.5g	27.1g	12g	41.7g	9.5g	1.3g

Serves: 2   **Prep time:** 5 minutes   **Cooking time:** 20 minutes
Ingredients:
- 40g reduced-fat Chorizo, sliced
- 2x150g cod fillets, or any white fish
- 1 medium red onion, peeled and finely chopped
- 1x400g can of chopped tomatoes
- 1 cloves of fresh smoked garlic clove, peeled and finely chopped
- 1 tsp smoked paprika
- freshly ground black pepper
- 1 tsp fresh parsley, to garnish
- 400g tin of mixed beans, drained

Instructions:
Preheat the oven to 190C

Cook the chorizo in a small pan for 2-3 minutes, then add the onion and garlic and fry gently until soft. Add the tomatoes, paprika, butter beans, and black pepper.

Bring to a simmer and cook for 10-15 mins or until slightly reduced and thickened.

In the mean time place the fish in an ovenproof dish and place in the oven, cook for 15 mins.

To serve divide the smokey beans between two warm plates and top each with a piece of fish and garnish with the parsley.

Butternut Squash Risotto

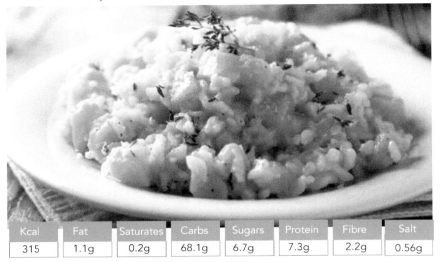

Kcal	Fat	Saturates	Carbs	Sugars	Protein	Fibre	Salt
315	1.1g	0.2g	68.1g	6.7g	7.3g	2.2g	0.56g

Serves: 4   **Prep time:** 10 minutes   **Cooking time:** 40 minutes

Ingredients:
- 1 tbsp Fage Total 0% Greek Yogurt
- 300g Arborio risotto rice
- 400g butternut squash, peeled de-seeded and cut into 2cm cubes
- 500ml warm fresh vegetable stock
- 1 large onion, peeled and finely chopped
- 2 garlic cloves, peeled and finely chopped
- freshly ground black pepper
- oil spray

Instructions:
Preheat the oven to 190C.

Spray a baking tray with the spray light, then place the butternut squash on top and spray with the oil spray again and bake for 20 minutes , remove and set aside when cooked.

Heat a large non-stick frying pan, and spray with spray light. Add the onions and garlic and cook until softened.

Now stir in the rice and cook for a further 3-4 minutes. Add a little of the stock, and when it has been absorbed by the rice add a little more until all the stock is absorbed.

Add the cooked butternut squash, and stir, then season with the freshly ground black pepper and cook for another 1 minute or so , remove from the heat and stir in the greek yogurt.

Serve immediately.

Sweet Potato and Okra Stew

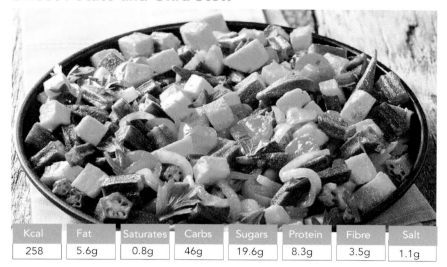

Kcal	Fat	Saturates	Carbs	Sugars	Protein	Fibre	Salt
258	5.6g	0.8g	46g	19.6g	8.3g	3.5g	1.1g

Serves: 1   **Prep time:** 5 minutes   **Cooking time:** 30 minutes
Ingredients:
- 150g sweet potatoes, peeled and cut into 1cm cubes
- 90g fresh okra, top and tailed and chopped into 1½cm slices
- 150ml vegetable stock
- 50g tomato passata
- 1 small onion, peeled and sliced
- 6 cherry tomatoes, halved
- 1 small red chilli, finely chopped
- 1 tsp garam masala
- ½ tsps turmeric
- Rapeseed oil spray

Instructions:
Heat a heavy-based frying pan and add a couple of sprays of the oil. Now add the onion, sweet potato and the red chilli and cook for 3-5 minutes, stirring occasionally.

Add the vegetable stock, garam masala, turmeric and tomato passata and cook for a further 10 minutes on a medium heat until the potatoes are just starting to soften.

Add the okra and the cherry tomatoes and simmer for a further 10 -12 minutes until the sauce has reduced right away.

Serve straight away – garnish with a few fresh parsley leaves (optional).

Cauliflower Rice

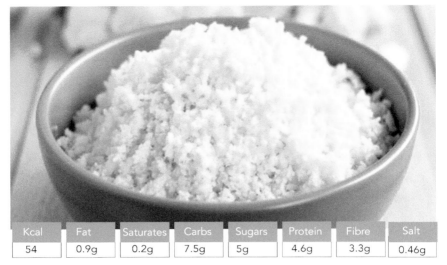

Kcal	Fat	Saturates	Carbs	Sugars	Protein	Fibre	Salt
54	0.9g	0.2g	7.5g	5g	4.6g	3.3g	0.46g

Serves: 1   **Prep time:** 5 minutes   **Cooking time:** 1 minute

Ingredients:
- 180g cauliflower florets
- 1 Knorr gluten-free and lactose free vegetable stock cube

Instructions:
Boil 1 litre of water in a saucepan, adding the vegetable stock cube.

Break the cauliflower into florets and whizz in a food processor until they form the consistency of breadcrumbs. Add this cauliflower 'rice' to the boiling water for 30 seconds, then drain well through a sieve before serving.

Egg Curry

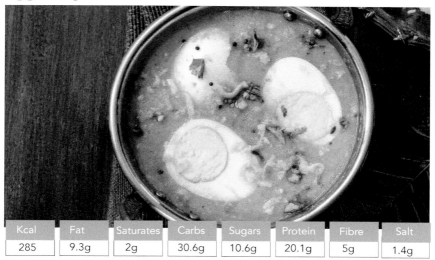

Kcal	Fat	Saturates	Carbs	Sugars	Protein	Fibre	Salt
285	9.3g	2g	30.6g	10.6g	20.1g	5g	1.4g

Serves: 2   **Prep time:** 5 minutes   **Cooking time:** 25 minutes

Ingredients:

- 3 medium eggs
- 1x400g tin of lentil soup
- 3 tsps garam masala or curry powder
- 2cm piece of fresh ginger root, grated, reserve some for garnish (optional)
- 1 red chilli, finely chopped
- 1 garlic clove, peeled and finely diced
- 1 large onion, peeled and finely diced
- 1x200g tin of chopped tomatoes
- 1 tbsp coriander, roughly chopped
- Rapeseed oil spray

Instructions:

Bring a pan of water to the boil and add the eggs, and cook for 3-4 minutes. Once cooked just set aside.

Heat a heavy-based large saucepan and spray with the oil spray. Add the onion, garlic, ginger and chilli cook gently until softened.

Add the garam masala or curry powder, tomatoes and lentil soup to the onion, garlic, ginger and chilli mix. Stir and reduce to a simmer. Cook for 15-20 minutes until the sauce has thickened

Carefully peel the eggs, and then cut in half. Transfer the curry sauce to a serving bowl and add the egg halves. Top with the chopped fresh coriander and a little grated fresh ginger (optional) and serve straight away.

Chickpea and Apricot Tagine

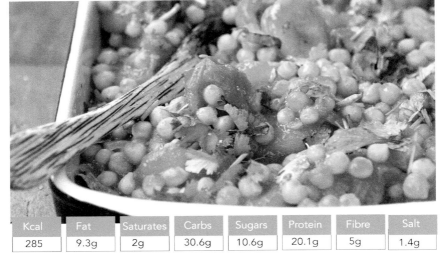

Kcal	Fat	Saturates	Carbs	Sugars	Protein	Fibre	Salt
285	9.3g	2g	30.6g	10.6g	20.1g	5g	1.4g

Serves: 2   **Prep time:** 5 minutes   **Cooking time:** 25 minutes

Ingredients:
- 1–3 tsps Lactose and gluten free vegetable stock powder
- 2 garlic cloves, crushed
- 1 piece (2cm) fresh ginger, chopped
- 1 tsp ground cumin
- 150g dried apricots
- 1 tbsp tomato puree
- 2 large onions, sliced
- 2x400g cans chickpeas, drained
- 1 tsp ground coriander
- 2x400g cans chopped tomatoes
- 2 tbsps golden syrup or honey
- fresh coriander, to serve

Instructions:
In a non-stick pan, dry-fry the onion and garlic until soft. Add the remaining ingredients and simmer gently for 30 minutes until the sauce has reduced and the apricots are soft.

Just before serving stir in the freshly chopped coriander.

TIP
Simmer over a long time to release the flavours or make the day before and chill overnight for a fuller flavour.

Spicy Prawn and Courgette Rice

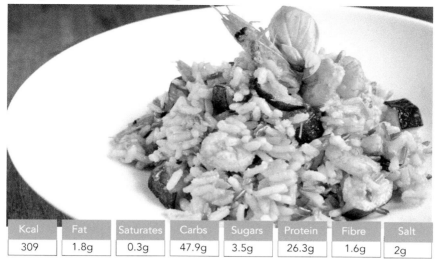

Kcal	Fat	Saturates	Carbs	Sugars	Protein	Fibre	Salt
309	1.8g	0.3g	47.9g	3.5g	26.3g	1.6g	2g

Serves: 1   **Prep time:** 5 minutes   **Cooking time:** 20 minutes
Ingredients:

- Rapeseed oil spray
- 1 tsp tomato puree
- 120g cooked king prawns
- 55g basmati and wild rice mix or plain basmati rice (dry weight)
- 1 medium courgette, cut into quarters,then cut into chunks about 1cm thick
- ½ tsps chilli flake
- salt and freshly ground black pepper

Instructions:
Heat a pan of water until boiling and add the rice, wild rice (optional) and chilli flakes. Cook for 15 minutes or until it has fully cooked. Once cooked drain the rice, but keep 2-3 tablespoons of the cooking liquid in reserve.

Heat a frying pan and add a couple sprays of rapeseed oil and add the courgettes. Cook for 3-5 minutes until they are starting to soften.

Add the rice, reserved cooking liquid, tomato puree and prawns to the frying pan. Reduce the heat slightly and stir all of the ingredients together. Cook for a further 2-3 minutes until the prawns are hot and the cooking liquor has been absorbed. Season with a little salt and pepper and add a few extra chilli flakes if you want to increase the spice. Serve immediately.

Minced Beef and Potato Hash

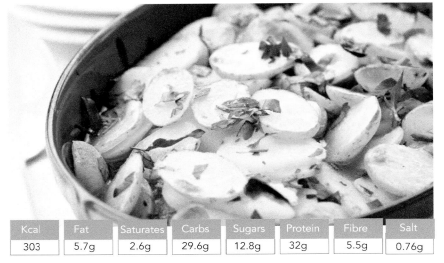

Kcal	Fat	Saturates	Carbs	Sugars	Protein	Fibre	Salt
303	5.7g	2.6g	29.6g	12.8g	32g	5.5g	0.76g

Serves: 1   **Prep time:** 10 minutes   **Cooking time:** 25 minutes

Ingredients:
- 120g lean minced beef
- ½ tsps stock powder
- ½ small red onion, diced
- 1x200g can chopped tomatoes
- 1 tsp tomato puree
- 120g cooked new potatoes
- salt and black pepper, to taste
- 1 tsp freshly chopped basil
- fresh flat-leaf parsley, to serve

Instructions:
Preheat the oven to 200°C, 400°F, Gas Mark 6.

Preheat a non-stick pan and dry-fry the mince and onion for 2-3 minutes. Add the tomatoes, puree,basil and stock powder, bringing it up to the boil. Simmer for 20 minutes. Pour into a small ovenproof dish.

Slice the potatoes and layer on top, lightly spraying with oil spray. Oven bake for 10 minutes to brown. Just before serving, sprinkle with flat leaf parsley. Serve with additional vegetables.

Lemon Chicken with Fine Green Beans

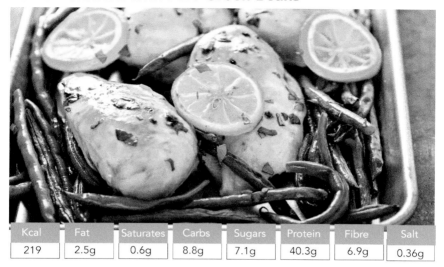

Kcal	Fat	Saturates	Carbs	Sugars	Protein	Fibre	Salt
219	2.5g	0.6g	8.8g	7.1g	40.3g	6.9g	0.36g

Serves: 4   **Prep time:** 5 minutes   **Cooking time:** 40 minutes

Ingredients:
- 800g frozen fine green beans
- 4x150 skinless and boneless chicken breasts
- salt and freshly ground black pepper
- 1 tsp flat-leaf parsley, chopped (optional)
- 2 tsps honey
- 2 lemons

Instructions:
Preheat the oven to 180C/160C fan/gas mark 4.

Add the juice of one lemon and honey to a bowl and mix well.

Use a large ovenproof dish or deep baking tray, and line it with the frozen fine green beans.

Place the chicken breasts on top of the fine green beans and brush each chicken fillet with the lemon and honey marinade, drizzling over the remaining marinade.

Season with the salt and black pepper. Slice the remaining lemon and scatter over the lemon slices and cover the dish with foil, shiny side down. Place in the oven and bake for 30 minutes.

Increase the oven temperature to 200C/180C fan/ gas mark 6. Remove the foil from the dish and return the chicken to the oven for a further 5-10 minutes until golden brown on top.

Serve hot with a little flat-leaf parsley over the top (optional).

Miso Honey Quorn Fillets with Mixed Peppers

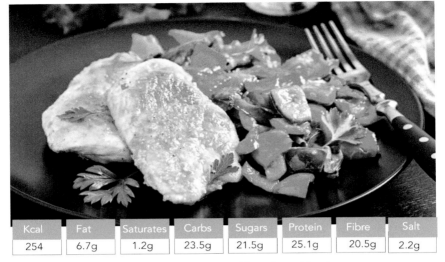

Kcal	Fat	Saturates	Carbs	Sugars	Protein	Fibre	Salt
254	6.7g	1.2g	23.5g	21.5g	25.1g	20.5g	2.2g

Serves: 1   **Prep time:** 5 minutes   **Cooking time:** 15 minutes

Ingredients:

- 150g Quorn Meat Free Fillets
- 1 large green pepper, de-seeded and diced
- 1 large red pepper, de-seeded and diced
- 1 ½ tsps white miso paste
- 1 tsp honey or golden syrup
- 1 tsp white wine vinegar
- Rapeseed oil spray

Instructions:

Place the miso paste and white wine vinegar with the honey and 1 tablespoon of water into a bowl and mix to make a marinade. Add the Quorn fillets and gently toss until completely coated in the mix. Set aside.

Heat a medium-sized non-stick frying pan and spray lightly with the rapeseed oil. Add the chunks of red and green pepper and gently fry for 3-4 minutes.

Make a space in the middle of the frying pan and add the marinated Quorn fillets. Reduce the heat slightly and cook for the Quorn fillets for 5 minutes on each side. Transfer to a warmed plate and serve.

Tomato and Basil Mushrooms

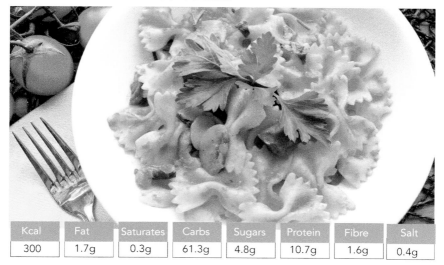

Kcal	Fat	Saturates	Carbs	Sugars	Protein	Fibre	Salt
300	1.7g	0.3g	61.3g	4.8g	10.7g	1.6g	0.4g

Serves: 2   **Prep time:** 5 minutes   **Cooking time:** 15 minutes

Ingredients:
- 350g cooked bow pasta
- 1 small red onion, chopped
- 125g chestnut mushrooms, sliced
- ½ vegetable stock cube, crumbled
- 2 fresh basil leaves, chopped
- 120g tomato passata

Instructions:

In a preheated non-stick pan, dry-fry the mushrooms and onion until soft.

Add the cumbled vegetable stock cube along with the tomato passata. Stir in the chopped basil.

Serve with the cooked pasta.

Aubergine, Courgette and Tomato Bake

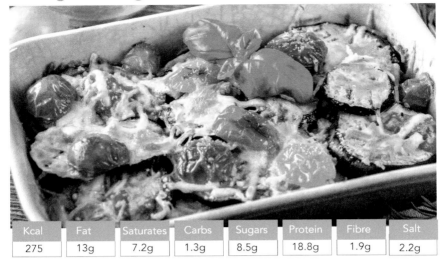

Kcal	Fat	Saturates	Carbs	Sugars	Protein	Fibre	Salt
275	13g	7.2g	1.3g	8.5g	18.8g	1.9g	2.2g

Serves: 1   **Prep time:** 10 minutes   **Cooking time:** 40 minutes

Ingredients:
- 50g low-fat cheese or vegan style cheddar, grated
- salt and freshly ground black pepper
- 160ml hot vegetable stock
- 100g mixed coloured cherry tomatoes, halved
- 1 medium courgette, top removed and sliced
- 1 medium aubergine, top removed and cut to 1 cm slices

Instructions:
Preheat the the oven to 200C,Gas mark 6, or use the baking oven in an Aga or similar

Layer the aubergine, courgettes and tomato halves in a small casserole dish. Pour over the hot vegetable stock and season with a little salt and freshly ground black pepper.

Place in the oven and cook for 25 minutes. Carefully remove from the oven and sprinkle over the grated cheese. Return to the oven for a further 15 minutes or until the cheese is melted and golden. Remove from the oven and serve with warm crusty bread or as a side.

TIP
This will serve 2 people as a side, this can be eaten cold.

Mushroom Omelette

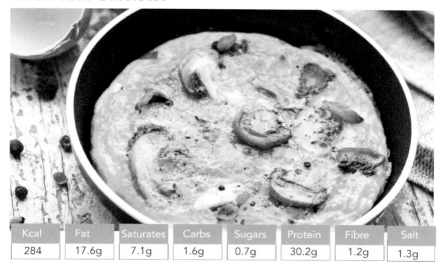

Kcal	Fat	Saturates	Carbs	Sugars	Protein	Fibre	Salt
284	17.6g	7.1g	1.6g	0.7g	30.2g	1.2g	1.3g

Serves: 1   **Prep time:** 10 minutes   **Cooking time:** 15 minutes

Ingredients:
- Rapeseed oil spray
- 2 eggs plus an additional 2 egg whites
- 100g mixed mushrooms, sliced
- 1 spring onion, root removed and finely sliced
- salt and pepper
- 30g low-fat mature cheese
- a couple of fresh basil leaves (optional) to serve

Instructions:

In a bowl beat the eggs and egg whites with a little salt and pepper.

Heat a heavy based frying pan and spray with spray oil. Add the onions and mushrooms and cook for 3-4 minutes or until softened.

Preheat a grill to medium heat.

Pour the egg mixture over the mushrooms, onions and sprinkle over the cheese. Cook for a further 3-4 minutes until almost set.

Place the frying pan under the grill for 2 minutes to finish off. Sprinkle over the basil leaves (optional).

Mixed Bean Vegetarian Chilli with Chocolate

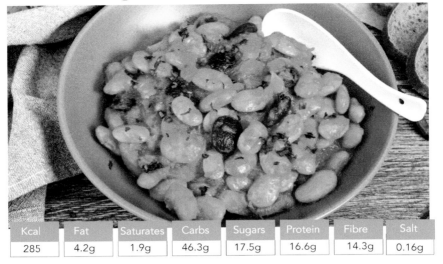

Kcal	Fat	Saturates	Carbs	Sugars	Protein	Fibre	Salt
285	4.2g	1.9g	46.3g	17.5g	16.6g	14.3g	0.16g

Serves: 4 **Prep time:** 5 minutes **Cooking time:** 25 minutes

Ingredients:
- 3x400g can mixed beans, rinsed and drained
- 1 large red onion, peeled and finely chopped
- 1 stick of celery, sliced
- 3 garlic cloves, peeled and finely chopped
- 2x400g can chopped tomatoes
- 2 red chillies, de-seeded and finely chopped
- 1 tbsp tomato puree
- 40g dark chocolate (70% cocoa) grated
- a pinch of sea salt
- freshly ground black pepper, to taste

Instructions:
Heat a large non-stick frying pan and dry fry the onion, chilli, celery and garlic, until softened.

Add the beans, tomatoes, puree and salt and simmer for 15 minutes. Stir in the grated chocolate and cook for a further 5 minutes.

Season with the black pepper and serve.

Mushroom and Lemon Quinoa Bake

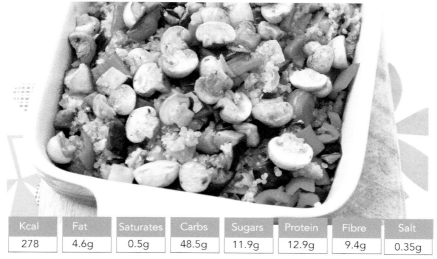

Kcal	Fat	Saturates	Carbs	Sugars	Protein	Fibre	Salt
278	4.6g	0.5g	48.5g	11.9g	12.9g	9.4g	0.35g

Serves: 2   **Prep time:** 20 minutes   **Cooking time:** 35 minutes

Ingredients:
- 180g chestnut mushrooms, halved
- 150g Quinoa, dry weight
- 750ml Lactose and gluten free vegetable stock
- 1 red onion, chopped
- 1 red pepper, diced
- 1 lemon, juice and zest
- salt and black pepper
- ½ tsps cumin seeds

Instructions:
Preheat the oven to 200°C, 400°F, Gas Mark 6. Dry-fry the onion, cumin, pepper and mushrooms in a non-stick pan until soft.

Place the Quinoa in a saucepan, add the stock and vegetables along with the lemon zest and juice. Bring to the boil, reduce the heat and simmer gently for 20 minutes until the water has been absorbed.

Remove from the heat and spoon into an ovenproof dish. Bake in a preheated oven for 10 minutes to crisp the top. Serve.

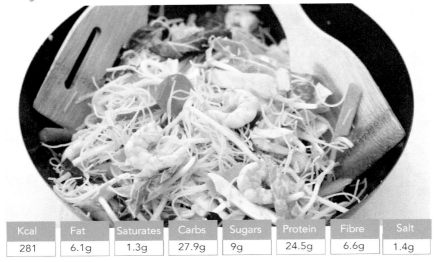

Kcal	Fat	Saturates	Carbs	Sugars	Protein	Fibre	Salt
281	6.1g	1.3g	27.9g	9g	24.5g	6.6g	1.4g

Serves: 4   **Prep time:** 10 minutes   **Cooking time:** 10 minutes

Ingredients:
- 400g raw king prawns
- 100g Tenderstem broccoli
- 100g thin asparagus
- Rapeseed oil spray
- black pepper, to taste
- 325g cooked rice noodles
- 2 tbsps light soy sauce
- 600g stir-fry vegetables
- 60ml rose wine
- 2 cloves of garlic, peeled and chopped
- 1 red onion, peeled and chopped

Instructions:
Heat a non-stick wok. Add a spray of oil and then stir-fry the onion, garlic, asparagus and broccoli for 2–3 minutes over medium heat, seasoning with black pepper.

Add the prawns and wine, and cook for 1–2 minutes to reduce the wine, before adding the stir-fry vegetables and soy sauce.

Add the noodles, stir well to combine with the rest of the ingredients and heat through, before serving.

TIP
If you don't want to use alcohol, add a little mango juice to sweeten this dish.

Broccoli and Cheese Pasta Bake

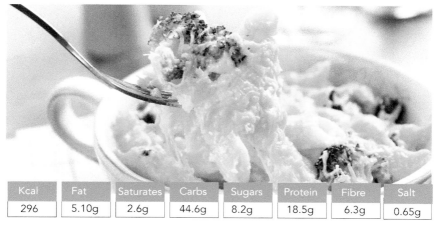

Kcal	Fat	Saturates	Carbs	Sugars	Protein	Fibre	Salt
296	5.10g	2.6g	44.6g	8.2g	18.5g	6.3g	0.65g

Serves: 4   **Prep time:** 5 minutes   **Cooking time:** 25 minutes

Ingredients:
- 250g broccoli spears
- 200g pasta shapes, dry weight
- 1 vegetable stock cube
- 200g low-fat soft cheese
- salt and black pepper, freshly ground
- 2 leeks, chopped
- 150ml semi-skimmed milk
- 1 tbsp fresh chives
- 30g reduced-fat or low-fat mature cheese, grated

Instructions:
Preheat the oven to 200C, 400F, Gas Mark 6.

Cook the pasta in a pan of water with the stock cube. Just before the pasta is cooked, add the broccoli and cook for 2 minutes.

Heat a non-stick pan and dry-fry the leeks for 1-2 minutes. Add the soft cheese and milk and stir well as the sauce thickens, adding more milk if required. Season with salt and pepper.

Drain the pasta and broccoli well and return to the pan. Stir in the cheese sauce, then pour into an ovenproof dish and top with the grated cheese and chives.

Bake in the oven for 10 minutes until golden brown.

If eating as a dinner, serve with a mixed salad or extra vegetables.

TIP
Spice up the sauce with a few dried chilli flakes.

Homemade Cauliflower Pizza Crust with Mozzarella and Basil

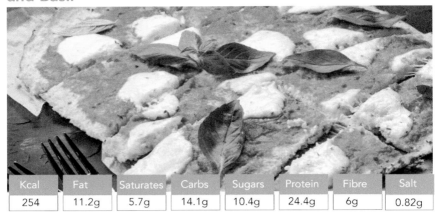

Kcal	Fat	Saturates	Carbs	Sugars	Protein	Fibre	Salt
254	11.2g	5.7g	14.1g	10.4g	24.4g	6g	0.82g

Serves: 2   **Prep time:** 5 minutes   **Cooking time:** 35 minutes

Ingredients:
- 500g frozen cauliflower florets, defrosted
- 125g reduced-fat mozzarella, sliced
- 1 medium sized tomato
- 40g tomato puree
- 1 small egg, beaten
- 40g reduced-fat cream cheese
- 1 tsp Italian dried herbs
- 1 pinch salt
- freshly ground black pepper

Instructions:
Pre-heat the oven to 200C, 400F, Gas Mark 6

Transfer the crumbed cauliflower to a clean tea-towel and wring out the excess fluid from the cauliflower and transfer the 'dry' cauliflower crumb to a mixing bowl. Add the beaten egg, cream cheese, herbs and pinch of salt to the mixing bowl and mix until evenly combined.

Line a baking tray with baking parchment or a silicone liner. Place the cauliflower mixture in the center of the baking tray and using a spoon shape the mixture into a large disc, making sure the thickness is about 5mm and a little thicker at the edges.

Bake for 20-25 minutes or until the pizza base is golden brown.
.
Whilst the pizza crust is baking de-seed the tomato and finely dice it. Place the diced tomato into a small bowl with the tomato puree, a little black pepper and 2 tsps water. Mix until a paste is formed and set aside until required.

Remove from the oven and carefully spread over the tomato paste and the mozzarella slices. Return to the oven and baked for a further 5-10 minutes. Serve with the fresh basil leaves sprinkled over the top.

Pork and Spring Vegetable Stir Fry

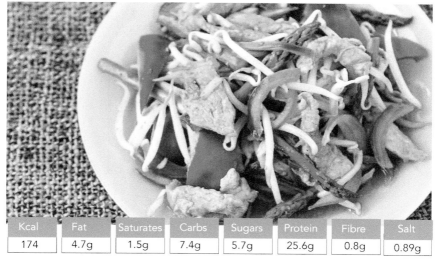

Kcal	Fat	Saturates	Carbs	Sugars	Protein	Fibre	Salt
174	4.7g	1.5g	7.4g	5.7g	25.6g	0.8g	0.89g

Serves: 1   **Prep time:** 10 minutes   **Cooking time:** 10 minutes

Ingredients:
- half a small red onion, peeled and sliced
- 100g pork fillets, cut into strips
- half a small green pepper, deseeded and sliced
- 45g bean sprouts
- 50g asparagus
- 1 tsp chilli sauce
- 1 tsp soy sauce
- black pepper
- juice and zest of 1 lime

Instructions:

Preheat a non-stick wok. Stir-fry the pork, onion and garlic for 3-4 minutes over a high heat, seasoning with pepper.

Add the remaining ingredients and toss well together, making sure all pieces of pork are cooked through. Serve on a warmed plate.

Keralan Style Fish Curry

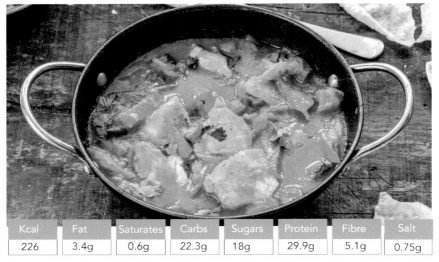

Kcal	Fat	Saturates	Carbs	Sugars	Protein	Fibre	Salt
226	3.4g	0.6g	22.3g	18g	29.9g	5.1g	0.75g

Serves: 2   **Prep time:** 5 minutes   **Cooking time:** 25 minutes

Ingredients:

- 280g firm white fish, boned and skin removed
- 1 red pepper, deseeded and diced
- 1 small red chilli, deseeded and finely diced
- 1 clove of garlic, peeled and finely chopped
- ½ tsps ground turmeric
- 1 tbsp curry powder
- ½ tsps mustard seeds
- 2cm piece of fresh ginger root, peeled and grated
- 1 small onion, peeled and chopped
- 1x200g can of chopped tomatoes
- 200ml coconut milk
- 1 tbsp fresh coriander, to serve (optional)

Instructions:

Cut the fish into chunks.

Heat a frying pan large pan and add a couple of sprays of the rapeseed oil, then add the mustard seeds and chopped red pepper and cook for 1-2 minutes.

Add the onion, garlic, grated ginger and chilli and cook for a further 2 minutes then add the curry powder and turmeric stir to combine the spices.

Add the coconut milk and chopped tomatoes, bring to the boil for 1 minute and then reduce the heat to a simmer. Add the fish and cook for a further 15 minutes until the fish has cooked and the sauce has thickened.

Add the fresh coriander and serve straight away.

Korean Aubergine Stew

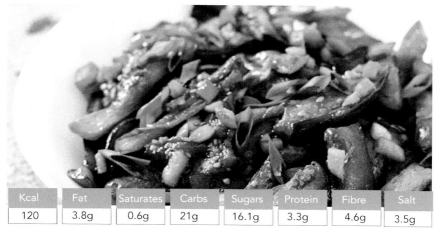

Kcal	Fat	Saturates	Carbs	Sugars	Protein	Fibre	Salt
120	3.8g	0.6g	21g	16.1g	3.3g	4.6g	3.5g

Serves: 2   **Prep time:** 5 minutes   **Cooking time:** 20 minutes
Ingredients:
- 1 medium onion
- 1 spring onion, cleaned, root removed and sliced - garnish
- Rapeseed oil spray
- 1 large aubergine

For the sauce:
- 2 tbsps soy sauce
- 2 tsps brown sugar
- 1 clove of garlic, peeled and finely diced
- 2cm piece of fresh ginger, finely grated
- ½ tsps sesame oil
- 1 tsp cornflour
- 1 red chilli, de-seeded and diced

Instructions:
In a small bowl, mix together all the sauce ingredients with 1 tablespoon of water.

Peel and slice your onion and cut the aubergine into thick strips about 1 to 2 cm wide and 4-5 cm long.

Heat a few sprays of the rapeseed oil in a frying pan over medium heat, then add the onion and gently fry for a few minutes until the onion softens and begins to brown. Now add the aubergine and then the sauce and stir to combine.

Cover and reduce the heat to a simmer and cook until the aubergine is tender and most of the liquid has been absorbed, stirring occasionally for about 10 minutes. If the aubergine starts to become a little dry whilst cooking, just add in a little more water.

Once cooked, serve straight away garnished with the chopped spring onion if using.

Garlic and Rosemary Chicken

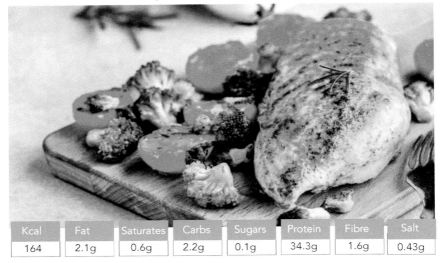

Kcal	Fat	Saturates	Carbs	Sugars	Protein	Fibre	Salt
164	2.1g	0.6g	2.2g	0.1g	34.3g	1.6g	0.43g

Serves: 2   **Prep time:** 5 minutes   **Cooking time:** 40 minutes

Ingredients:
- 2x140g skinless chicken breasts
- 2 large sprigs of fresh rosemary, broken down
- 2 garlic cloves
- salt and pepper, to season
- 200ml Knorr gluten-free and lactose free chicken stock

Instructions:
Heat a heavy based frying, then add the garlic and rosemary, cooking gently for 2-3 minutes.

Add the chicken breasts to the garlic and rosemary and fry until golden brown on both sides.

Add the chicken stock and bring to the boil, then turn the heat down to achieve a gentle simmer. Cook for 25 minutes.

To serve place the chicken on a warmed serving dish and pour over any remaining juices from the frying pan. Serve with a selection of vegetables.

Aubergine and Chickpea Stew

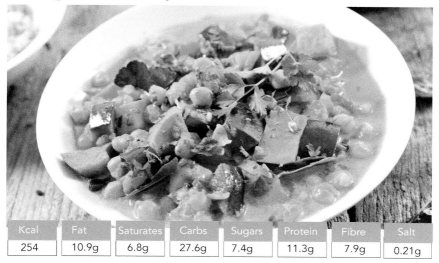

Kcal	Fat	Saturates	Carbs	Sugars	Protein	Fibre	Salt
254	10.9g	6.8g	27.6g	7.4g	11.3g	7.9g	0.21g

Serves: 4   **Prep time:** 25 minutes   **Cooking time:** 2 hours

Ingredients:

- 2 garlic cloves, chopped
- 1 large aubergine
- 1x180g sweet potato, peeled and cubed
- 1 tbsp ground coriander
- 1x400ml can reduced-fat coconut milk
- 2 tbsps basil, freshly chopped
- 2 red onions, diced
- 100g chestnut mushrooms, chopped
- 1 tbsp fresh ginger, peeled and finely chopped
- 1x210g can chickpeas, drained
- 50g red lentils
- coriander, to serve
- salt and black pepper, freshly ground
- 1 Lactose and gluten free vegetable stock cube, crumbled
- 1 tsp gluten free lemongrass paste

Instructions:

Preheat a non-stick wok or frying pan. Dry-fry the onion and garlic until soft and lightly coloured. Add the aubergine, sweet potatoes and mushrooms, browning for 4-5 minutes.

Transfer to a slow cooker and add the remaining ingredients. Simmer on a low setting for 2 hrs. Reduce the heat and allow to simmer gently as the sauce thickens.

Just before serving stir in the basil.

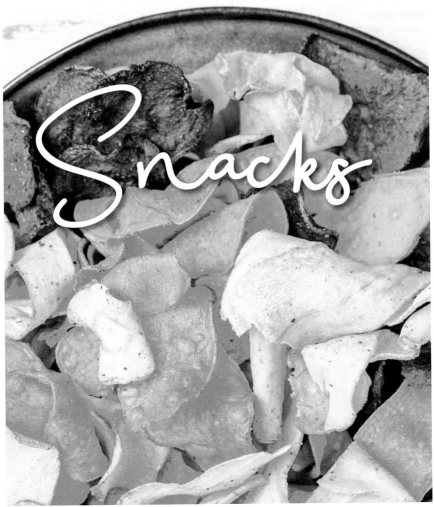

Snacks

Low-fat Oatcakes

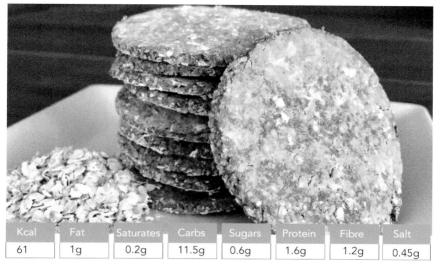

Kcal	Fat	Saturates	Carbs	Sugars	Protein	Fibre	Salt
61	1g	0.2g	11.5g	0.6g	1.6g	1.2g	0.45g

Serves: 10   **Prep time:** 5 minutes   **Cooking time:** 22 minutes

Ingredients:
- 120g porridge oats or gluten free porridge oats
- 30g wholemeal flour or gram flour
- 40g cooked and mashed sweet potato
- ¼ tsps sea salt
- ¼ tsps bicarbonate of soda
- 50ml hot water

Instructions:
Pre-heat the oven to 190C, 375F, gas mark 5

Mix together the oats, flour, salt, sugar and bicarbonate of soda in a clean mixing bowl then add the mashed sweet potato and rub together until everything is mixed and has the consistency of large bread crumbs.

Add the water (from a recently boiled kettle) bit by bit and combine until you have a thick dough, being careful as it will be hot. The amount of water may vary slightly depending on the oats and flour used.

Sprinkle some extra flour on a clean work surface and roll out the dough to approx. 3/4mm thickness using a 8cm round cutter cut out 10 discs.

Line a baking tray with baking parchment and place the oatcakes equally spaced on the tray. Bake for 20-22 minutes or until slightly golden brown in colour. Allow to cool and store in an airtight container for 3-4 days.

TIP
Use gram flour and gluten free porridge oats for a gluten free version.

Cocoa and Raisin Energy Balls

Kcal	Fat	Saturates	Carbs	Sugars	Protein	Fibre	Salt
85	4.4g	1.1g	8.7g	3.7g	2.6g	1.2g	0.07g

Makes: 18   **Prep time:** 5 minutes

Ingredients:
- 120g porridge oats
- 120g peanut butter
- 1 tbsp honey or golden syrup
- 2 tsp flaxseeds
- 2 tsp chia seeds
- 3 tsp dark cocoa powder
- 60g raisins
- ½ tsp vanilla extract

Instructions:
Place all of the ingredients in a large mixing bowl. Stir to combine.

If the mixture seems too wet, add a bit more oats. If it's too dry, add a bit more peanut butter. It should be a sticky dough that holds together.

Place the bowl in the refrigerator for 30 minutes to set.

Divide the mixture into 18 equal portions, and roll into balls, store in an airtight container in the fridge.

These will keep for 10-12 days in the fridge or they can be frozen for up to two months.

Courgette Bombs

Kcal	Fat	Saturates	Carbs	Sugars	Protein	Fibre	Salt
27	1.7g	0.7g	0.6g	0.5g	2.4g	0g	0.14g

Makes: 12   **Prep time:** 5 minutes **Cooking time:** 12-15 minutes

Ingredients:
- 400g courgettes, grated and excess water pressed out
- 2 medium eggs, beaten
- 25g pecorino cheese
- Pinch of black pepper

Instructions:
Preheat the oven to 200C, 400F, Gas Mark 6.

Place all of the ingredients into a bowl and gently mix together, until combined.

Divide into 12 portions, and shape into balls. Place on a baking tray lined with baking parchment and place in the oven, cook for 12-15 mins until they start to go golden brown.

Remove from the oven and carefully trim back any egg leakage. Eat hot or cold. These will keep in the fridge for 2-3 days.

Over-night Slow Roasted Tomatoes

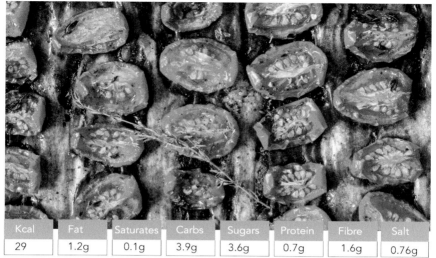

Kcal	Fat	Saturates	Carbs	Sugars	Protein	Fibre	Salt
29	1.2g	0.1g	3.9g	3.6g	0.7g	1.6g	0.76g

Serves: 4   **Prep time:** 5 minutes   **Cooking time:** 4 minutes

Ingredients:
- 500g ripe tomatoes
- Rapeseed oil spray
- Pinch sea salt
- 2 sprigs fresh thyme - optional

Instructions:
Pre-heat the oven to 220C, 475 F, Gas Mark 9.

Line a heavy baking tray with parchment.

Quarter the tomatoes and lay them skin side down on the baking tray in one even layer.

Spray lightly with the oil spray and sprinkle over the sea salt and fresh thyme if using.

Place them onto the top shelf in the oven and cook for 4 minutes, turn the oven off and leave the tomatoes to cook in the residual heat for at least 5-6 hours or ideally overnight.

When the tomatoes are cooked, transfer them to a plastic airtight container and store in the fridge.

They will keep for 4-5 days.

TIP
Amazing served in salads, in a tuna sandwich or just on their own as a quick snack.

Date and Nut Energy Balls

Kcal	Fat	Saturates	Carbs	Sugars	Protein	Fibre	Salt
99	7g	1g	5.6g	0.01g	2.8g	0.5g	0.01g

Makes: 8   **Prep time:** 5 minutes

Ingredients:
- 120g medjool dates, pitted
- 30g ground almonds
- 30g walnut halves
- 25g plain cashews
- 1 tsp chia seeds
- 1tsp flax seeds
- 1 ½ tsp dark cocoa powder
- ½ tsp vanilla extract

Instructions:
Place the walnuts, cashews, chia and flaxseeds in a food processor and blitz until a fine crumb.

Add the ground almonds and cocoa powder and blitz for a further 30 seconds.

Add the dates and the vanilla extract and blitz until it forms a sticky dough.

Dived the mixture into 8 portions and roll each portion into a ball and place on a tray covered in baking parchment.

Place them in the fridge for 30 minutes to set, then transfer to a plastic container and store in the fridge for up to 7 days.

Not suitable for freezing.

Posh Devilled Eggs

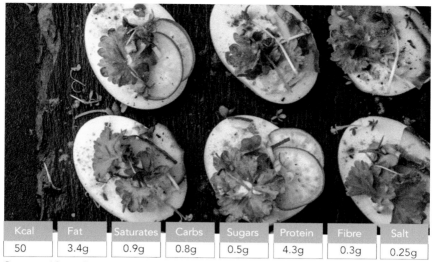

Kcal	Fat	Saturates	Carbs	Sugars	Protein	Fibre	Salt
50	3.4g	0.9g	0.8g	0.5g	4.3g	0.3g	0.25g

Serves: 12   **Prep time:** 10 minutes   **Cooking time:** 15 minutes

Ingredients:
- 6 large eggs
- 60g extra light mayonaise
- 1 pinch chilli powder
- ½ tsps smoked paprika
- ½ tsps English mustard
- a few fresh salad vegetables, such as radishes, cucumber, onion etc for garnish (optional)
- 1 tbsp mixed fresh herbs, such as parsley and coriander (optional)

Instructions:
Bring some water to the boil in a large saucepan then carefully add the eggs, one by one, into the pan and bring back to the boil. Boil for 4 minutes, then remove from the heat and allow to stand for 6 minutes.

Place the eggs into a large bowl of iced water, and allow to cool for 5-10 minutes. Then carefully removed and discard the shell. Using a sharp knife cut the eggs in half lengthways.

Carefully scoop out the yolk from each half and place in a bowl with the mayonnaise, mustard, 1/4 tsp smoked paprika, chilli powder and 1tsp of cold water. Beat the mixture until thick and smooth. Using a teaspoon divide the mixture equally between the 12 egg halves.

Sprinkle over the remaining smoked paprika and garnish with the fresh herbs and vegetables if using. Serve straight away or store in the fridge for 4 hours.

Cloud Bread

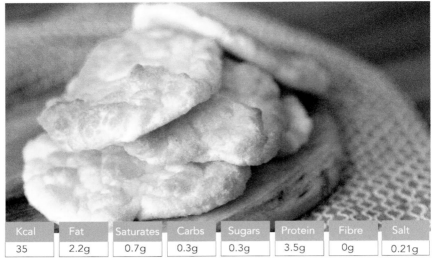

Kcal	Fat	Saturates	Carbs	Sugars	Protein	Fibre	Salt
35	2.2g	0.7g	0.3g	0.3g	3.5g	0g	0.21g

Serves: 6   **Prep time:** 5 minutes   **Cooking time:** 15 minutes

Ingredients:
- 1 pinch salt
- 30g low-fat cream cheese
- 2 large eggs, separated

Instructions:
Preheat the oven to 200C, 400F, Gas Mark 6.

Place the egg whites into a clean bowl and whisk until they are firm peaks, then add the salt and whisk for a further 10 seconds.

Place the egg yolks and cream cheese into a separate bowl and whisk for 1 minute until smooth. Gently fold the cream cheese and egg yolk mixture into the whisked egg whites, keeping as much air in the egg whites as possible.

Line a baking tray with baking parchment or similar. Make six equal mounds of the mixture on the tray, and spread out gently with the back of a spoon until they are about 1cm in thickness.

Bake in the oven for 12-15 minutes or until they are golden brown. Remove from the oven and allow to cool for 1-2 minutes, then carefully remove from the tray and allow to cool completely. Store in an airtight container at room temperature for 2-3 days.

Kale Crisps

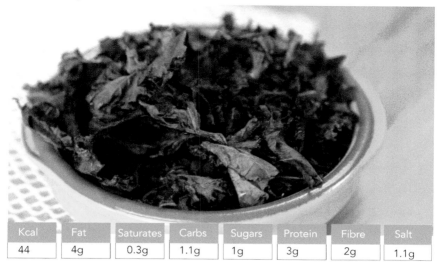

Kcal	Fat	Saturates	Carbs	Sugars	Protein	Fibre	Salt
44	4g	0.3g	1.1g	1g	3g	2g	1.1g

Serves: 1   **Prep time:** 3 minutes   **Cooking time:** 10 minutes

Ingredients:
- 80g kale
- Rapeseed oil spray
- salt
- 0.25 tsps cumin seed, optional

Instructions:
Pre-heat the oven to 180C, 350F, gas mark 4

Scatter the kale over a baking tray, sprinkle over the cumin seeds if using and then a couple of sprays of the rapeseed oil and season with a little salt.

Bake in the oven for 9-10 minutes, or until they have just gone crispy. Be careful as they will burn very quickly if you don't watch them.

Remove from the oven, allow to cool. These will keep in an airtight container for 24 hours.

Spiced Baked Chickpeas

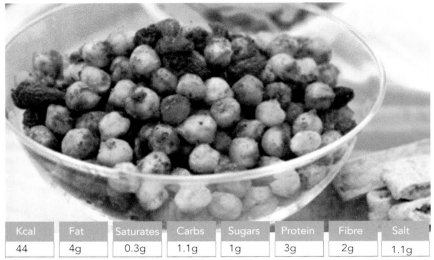

Kcal	Fat	Saturates	Carbs	Sugars	Protein	Fibre	Salt
44	4g	0.3g	1.1g	1g	3g	2g	1.1g

Serves: 1   **Prep time:** 3 minutes   **Cooking time:** 10 minutes

Ingredients:
- 1 tbsp soft brown sugar
- 2 tbsps raisins
- 1x400g can chickpeas
- 1 tbsp garam masala
- cayenne pepper

Instructions:
Preheat the oven to 200C, 400F, Gas Mark 6.

Drain the can of chickpeas well and place on a non-stick baking tray.

Mix together 1 tbsp Garam masala and 1 tbsp soft brown sugar and sprinkle over the chickpeas and bake in the oven for 20 minutes.

Dust with cayenne pepper and serve in bowls mixed with 2 tbsps raisins.

TIP
Serve these spicy low-fat treats warm.

Sweet Potato Crisps

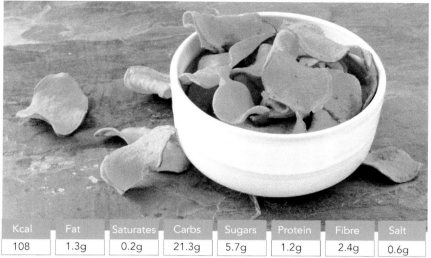

Kcal	Fat	Saturates	Carbs	Sugars	Protein	Fibre	Salt
108	1.3g	0.2g	21.3g	5.7g	1.2g	2.4g	0.6g

Serves: 2   **Prep time:** 5 minutes   **Cooking time:** 10 minutes

Ingredients:
- 200g sweet potato
- 1 pinch sea salt
- Rapeseed oil spray

Instructions:
Wash the sweet potato, and pat dry – do not peel. Pre-heat the oven to 210C, 415F, Gas mark 7

Slice into very fine slices using a vegetable peeler or mandolin onto kitchen paper to absorb any moisture. Cover with kitchen paper and pat well.

Lay out in a single layer on a non-stick baking tray. Season with a pinch of salt and lightly spray with oil spray. Bake in the oven for 8-10 minutes until crisp

Remove from the oven and cool on a wire rack. When cold place in bowls and serve.

Recipe Index

Fried Egg with Spinach and Tomatoes 94
Garlic and Rosemary Chicken 146
Griddled Chicken with Wedges and Roasted Tomatoes 123
Ham Salad Bagel 76
Homemade Cauliflower Pizza Crust with Mozzarella and Basil 142
Honey and Thyme Baked Salmon 110
Indian Style Roasted Cauliflower Steak 104
Kale Crisps 155
Keralan Style Fish Curry 144
Korean Aubergine Stew 145
Leek, Mushroom and Pepper Pasta 100
Leftover Chicken Noodle Soup 86
Lemon Chicken with Fine Green Beans 133
Low-fat Oatcakes 149
Melon, Prosciutto and Olive Salad 99
Minced Beef and Potato Hash 132
Miso Honey Quorn Fillets with Mixed Peppers 134
Mixed Bean Vegetarian Chilli with Chocolate 138
Mixed Frozen Berry Smoothie 65
Mushroom and Lemon Quinoa Bake 139
Mushroom and Marmite Spaghetti 122
Mushroom Crumpet 57
Mushroom Frittata 66
Mushroom Omelette 137
Mushrooms in a Creamy Tarragon Sauce 78
Naan Bread Chicken and Pepper Pizza 120
Oat, Banana and Cinnamon Breakfast Cookies 60
Open Egg and Prawn Sandwich 71
Over-night Slow Roasted Tomatoes 151
Pan Fried Salmon on a Bed of Wilted Spinach 114
Pasta with Pea and Mint Pesto 74
Pearl Couscous Salad 90
Pomegranate, Chickpea and Tomato Couscous Salad 84
Pork and Spring Vegetable Stir Fry 143
Posh Devilled Eggs 153
Puy Lentil and Pearl Couscous Vegetable Salad 96
Quick Bacon Spaghetti Carbonara 124
Quick Frozen Veg Pizza 111

Quick Mushroom Pate 107

Rich Sausage and Mushroom Casserole 117

Savoury Egg, Mushroom and Spinach Porridge 80

Scrambled and smoked Salmon on a Toasted Bread Roll 73

Scrambled Egg and Mushrooms on Bread 70

Simple Minestrone Soup 85

Simple Zesty Chicken Salad 75

Smoked Cod with Rice and Red Peppers 113

Spiced Baked Chickpeas 156

Spicy Beans with Mushrooms 98

Spicy Prawn and Courgette Rice 131

Strawberry and Cottage Cheese Crispbreads 79

Strawberry Muesli Mix 64

Stuffed Aubergine with Red Lentils 121

Super Easy Broccoli Soup 87

Sweet Potato and Okra Stew 127

Sweet Potato Crisps 157

Three Pepper Frittata 68

Tomato and Basil Mushrooms 135

Tuna Pate 97

Tuna Salad Lettuce Wraps 89

Tzatziki Style Crispbreads 88

Vegan and Dairy Free Breakfast Smoothie 57

Vegetarian Stuffed Peppers 105

Zesty Crayfish and Rocket Sandwich 81